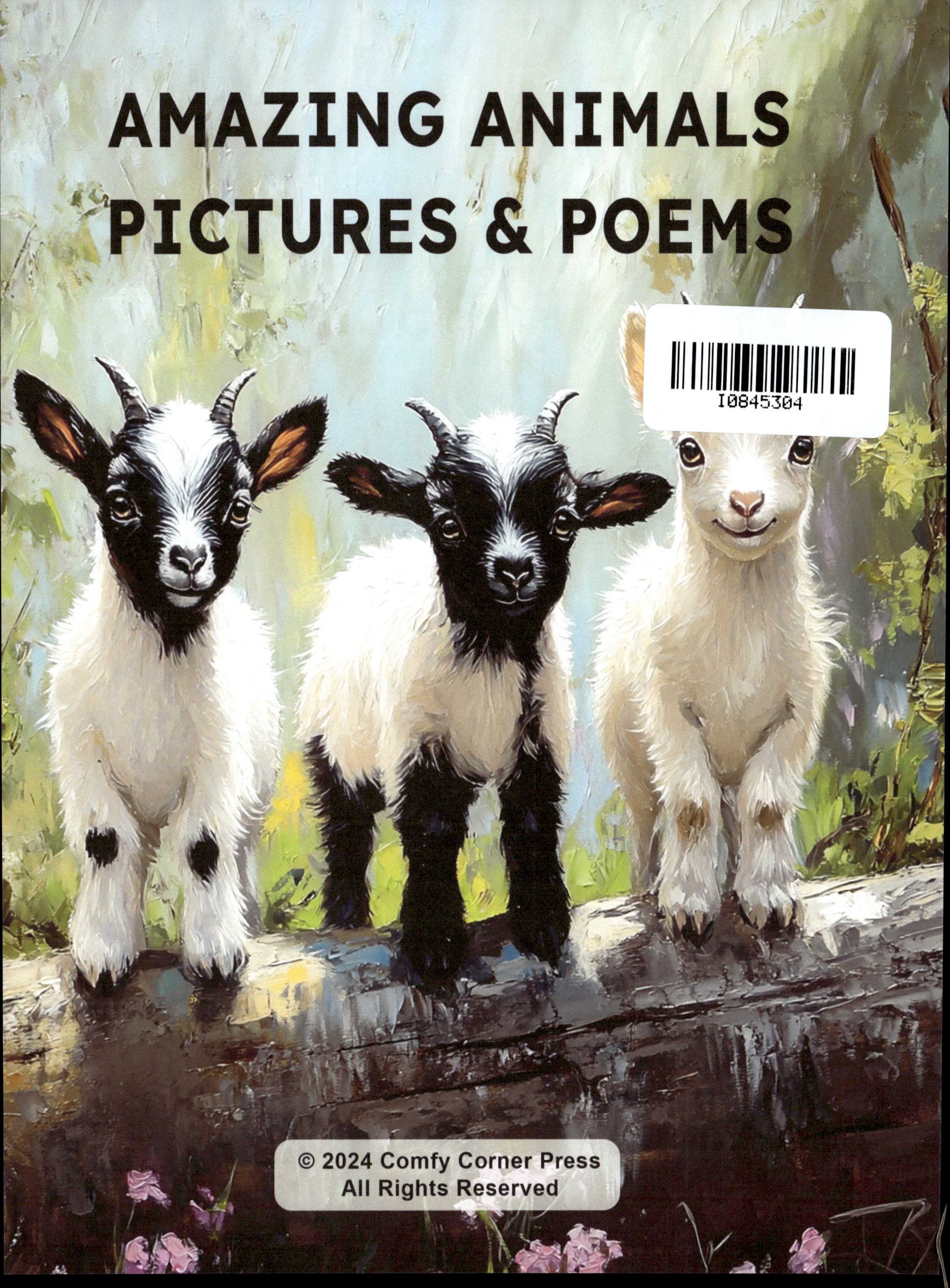

AMAZING ANIMALS
PICTURES & POEMS
I0845304
© 2024 Comfy Corner Press
All Rights Reserved

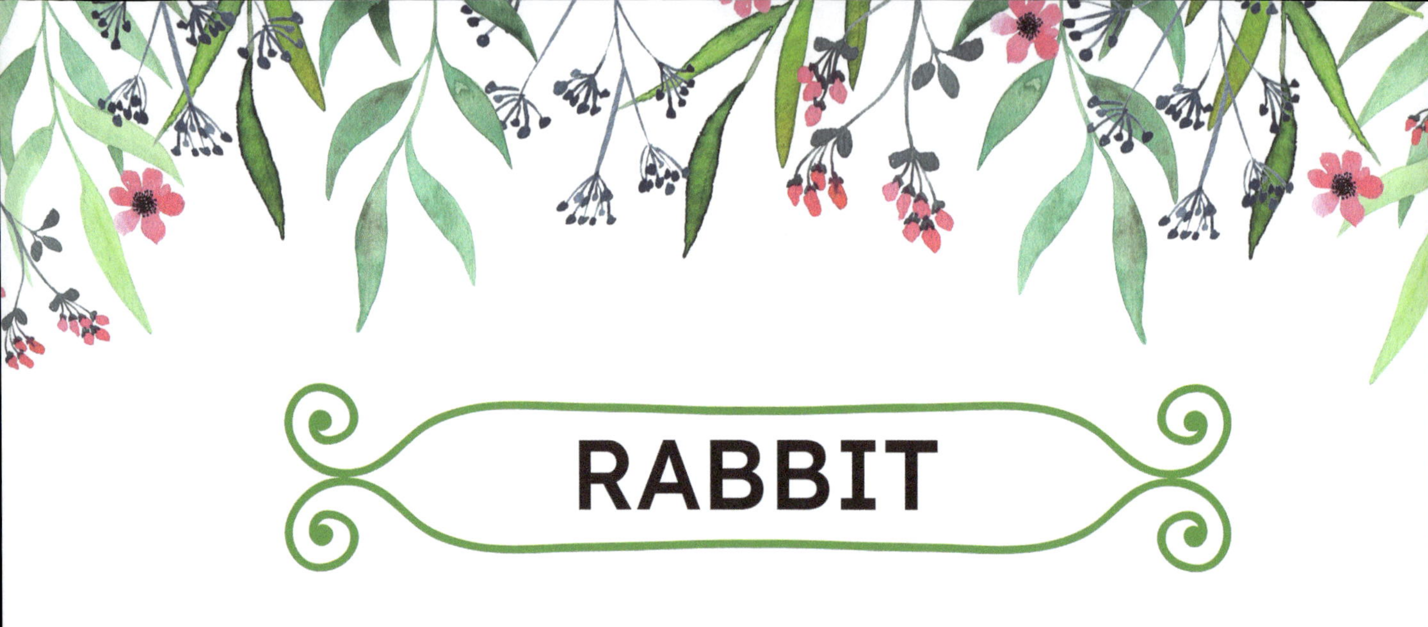

RABBIT

A bunny rabbit, soft and small,

Hops through meadows in the fall.

With twitching nose and ears so tall,

He's the cutest of them all!

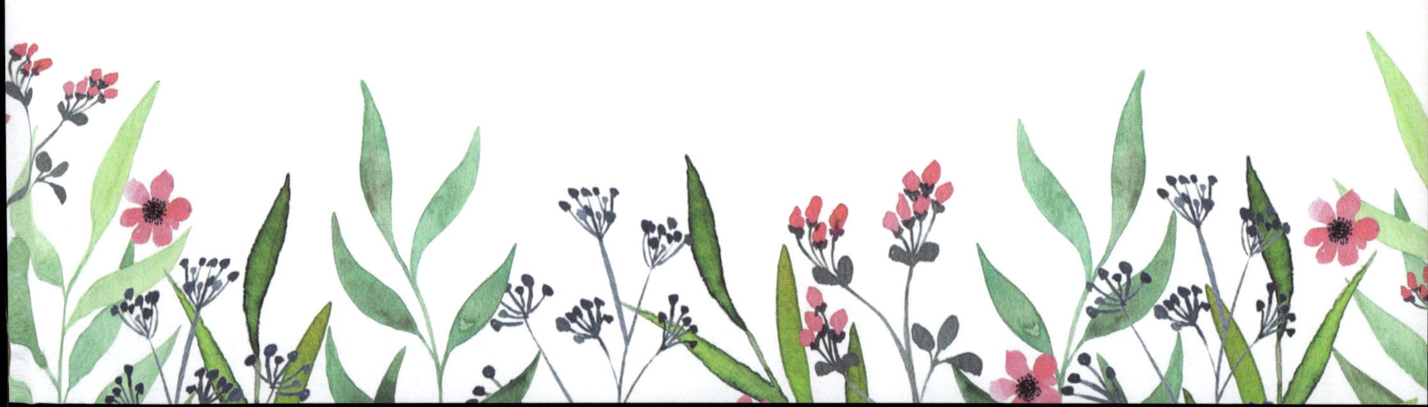

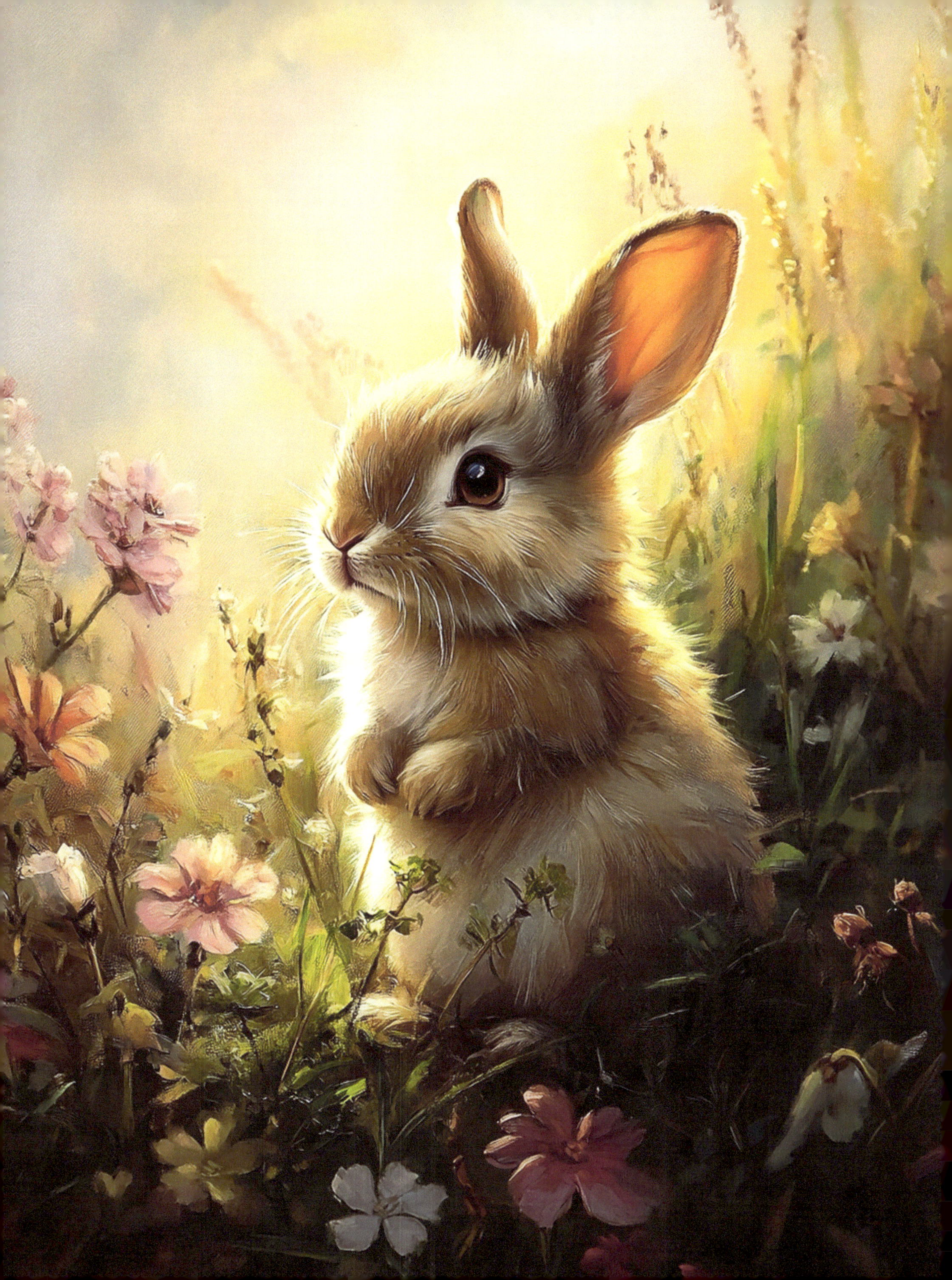

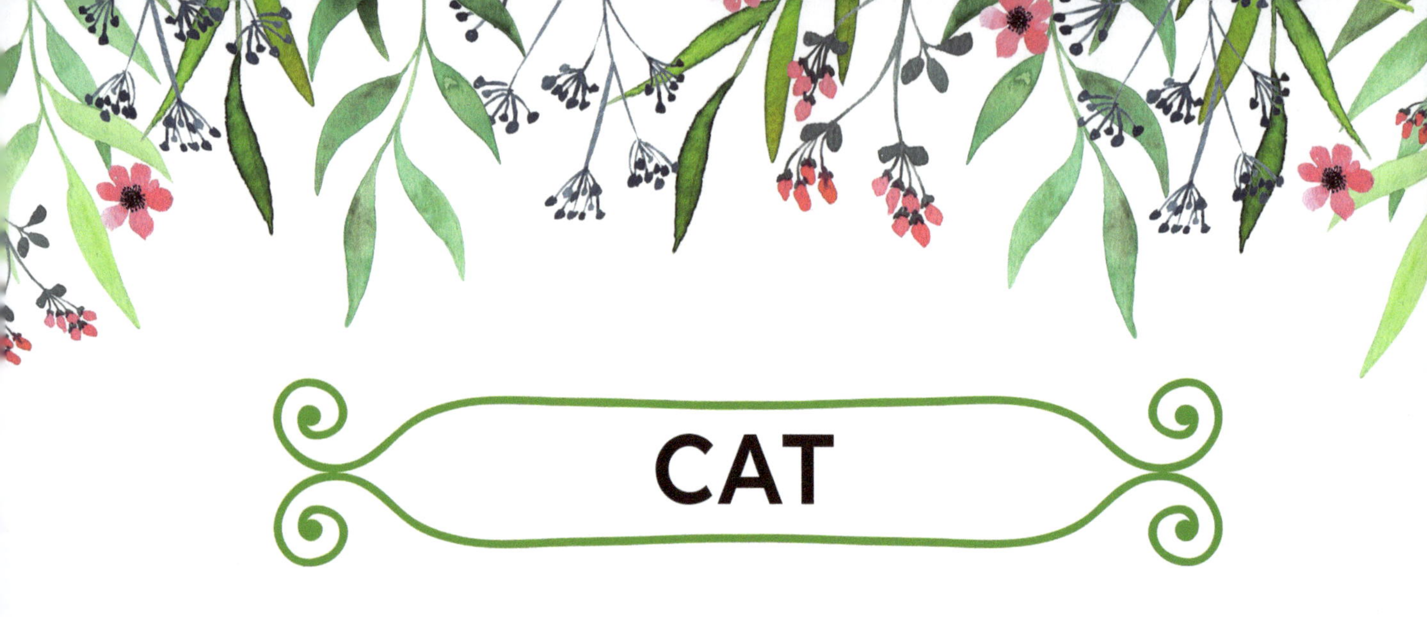

CAT

A tabby cat with eyes of green,

Perches on a wall, unseen.

Watching all the world go by,

A tiny tiger 'neath the sky.

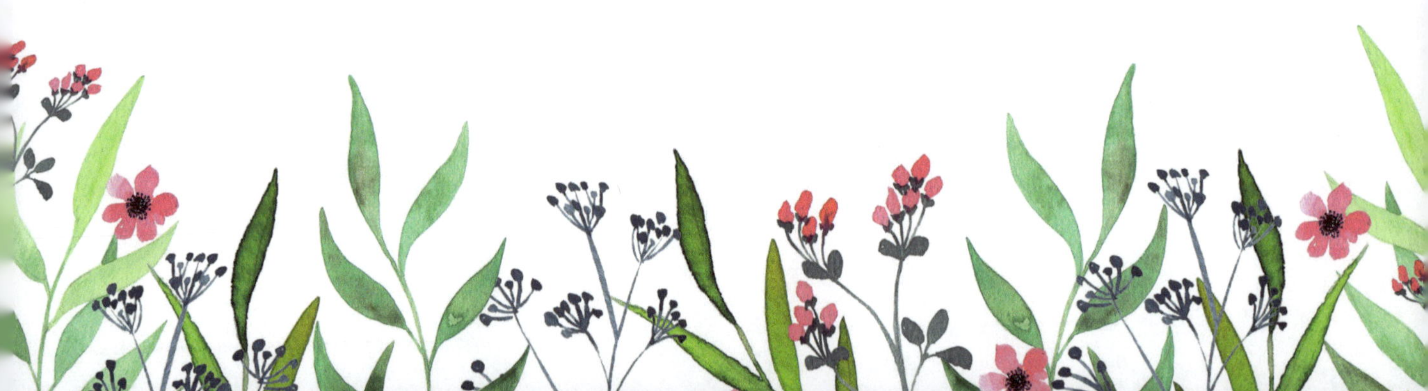

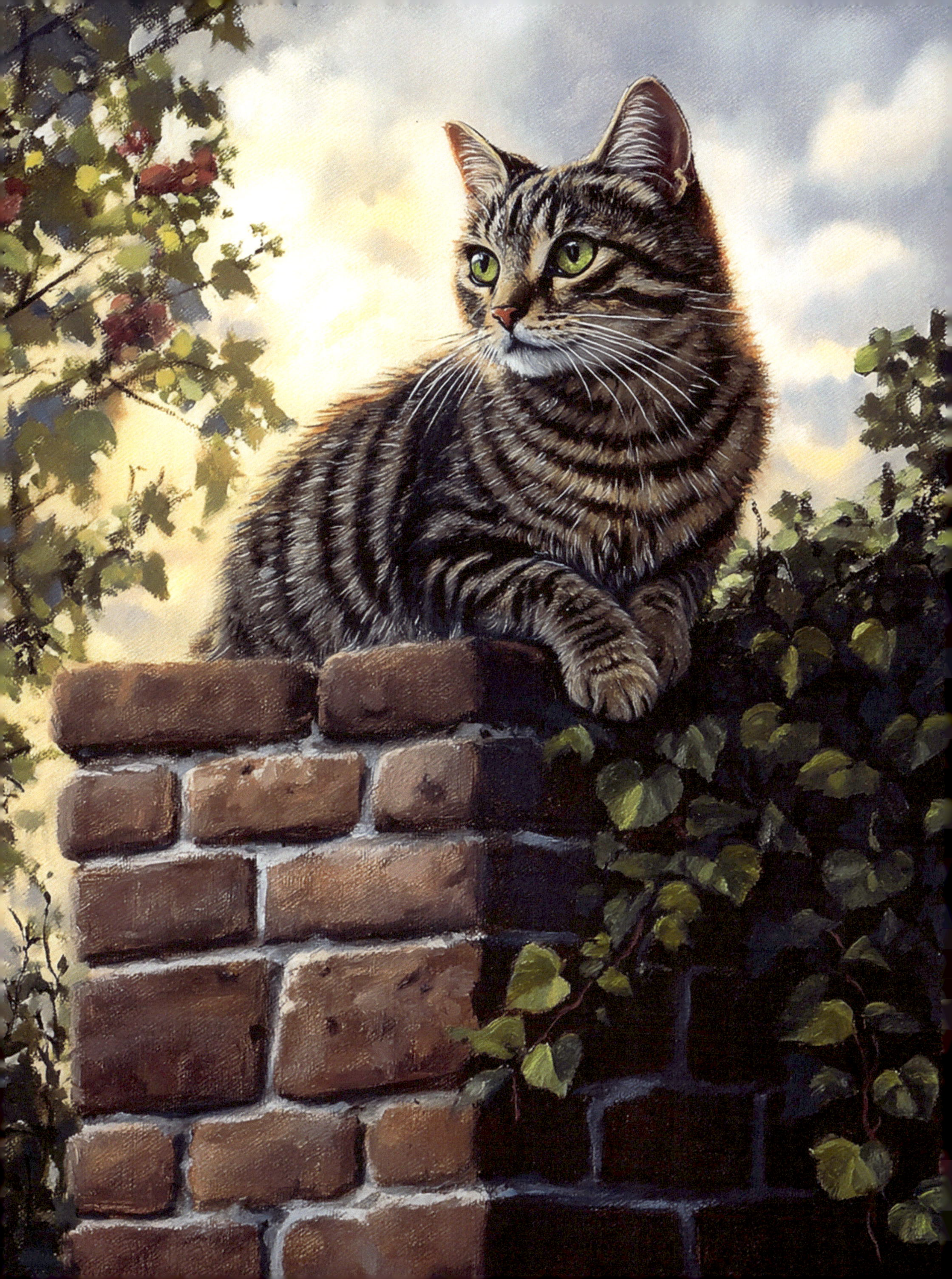

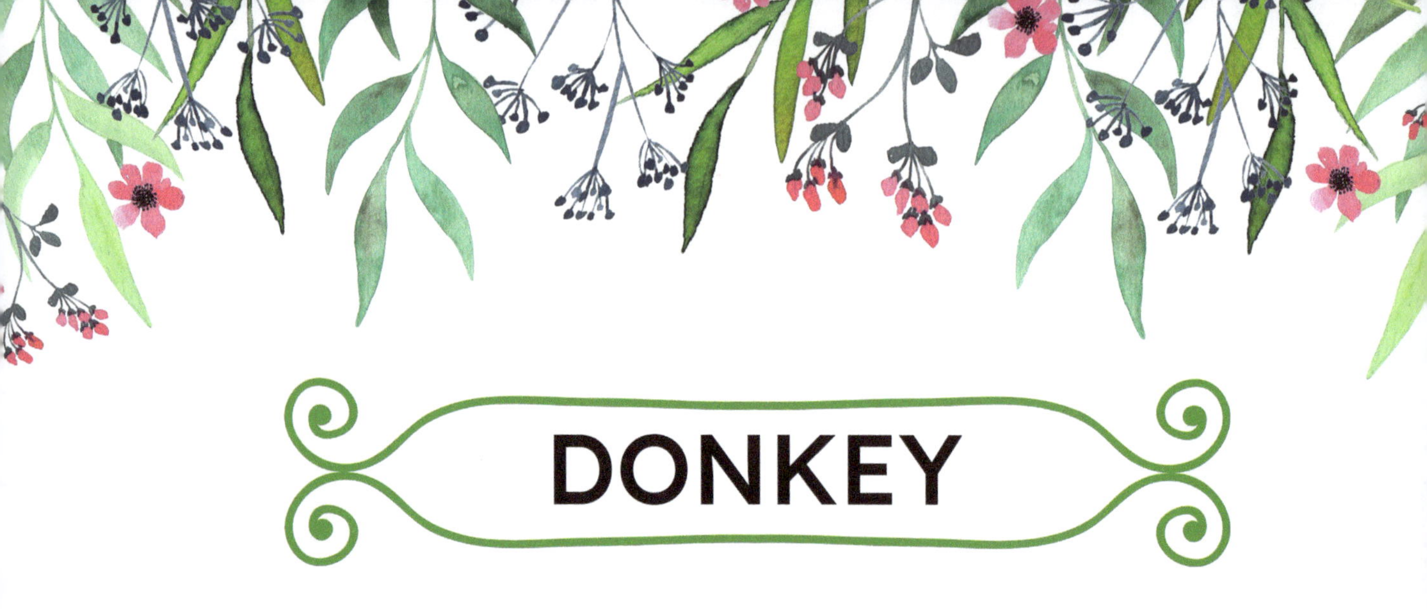

DONKEY

Under the shade of a leafy tree,

A donkey stands, sweet as can be.

Braying gently in the summer air,

The sweetest friend without a care.

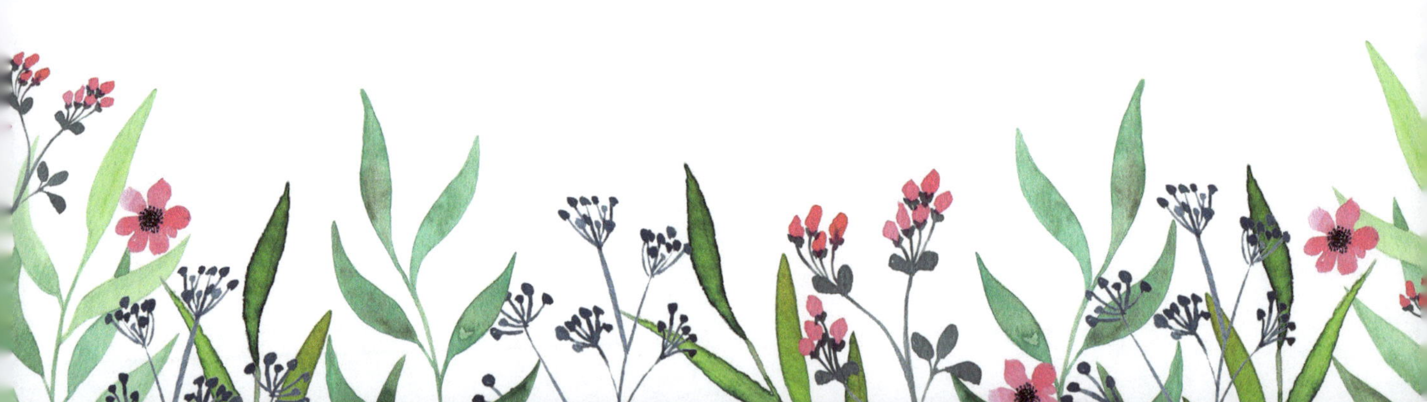

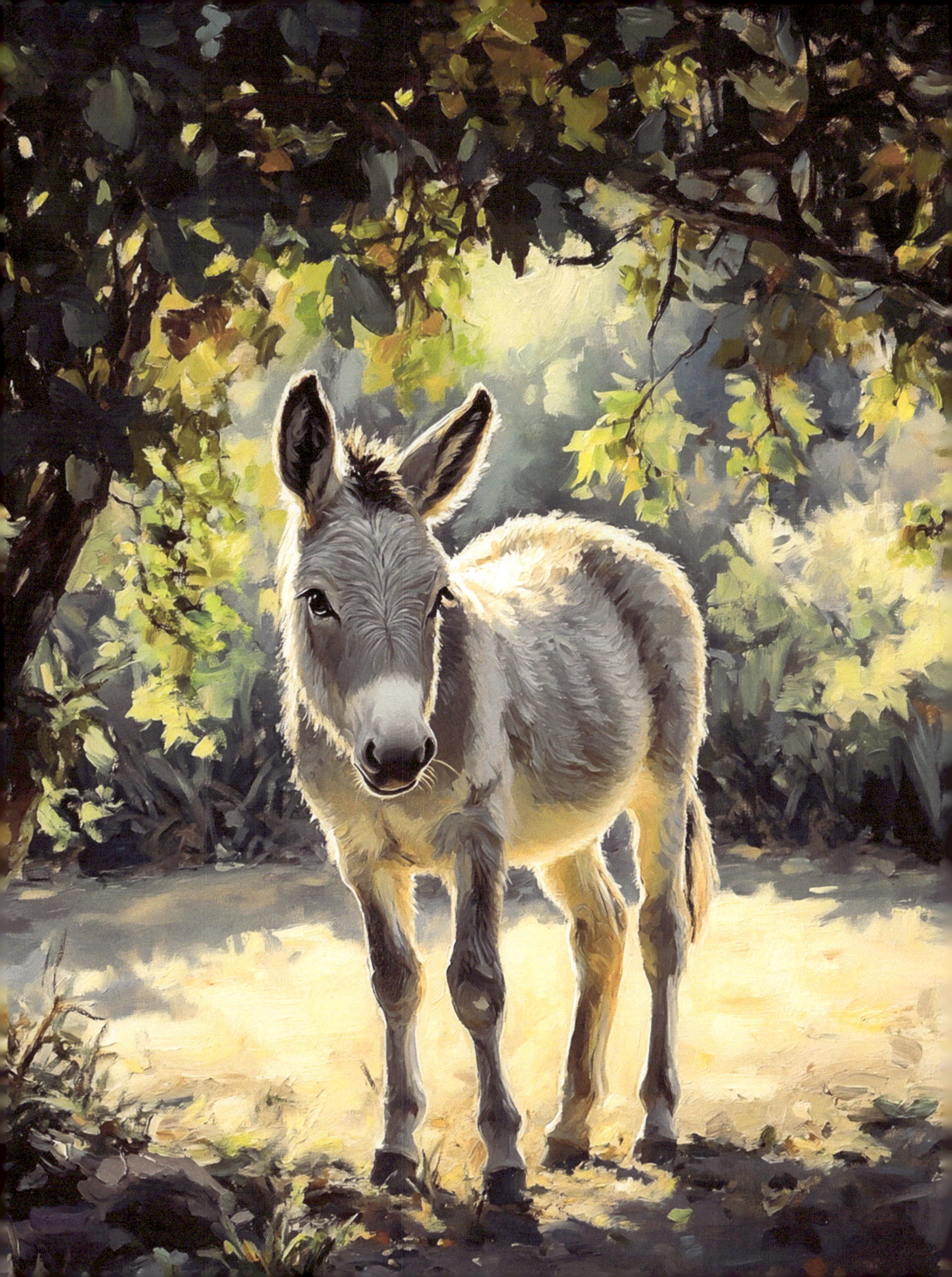

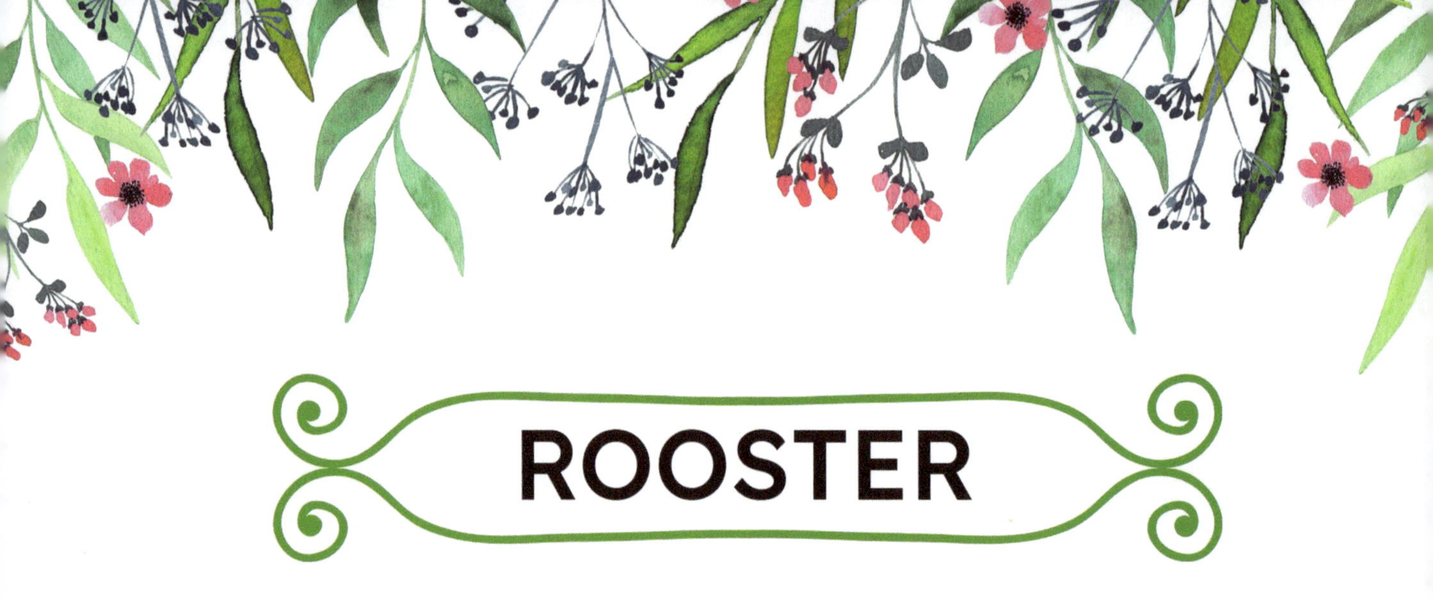

ROOSTER

A Rhode Island Red with feathers bright,

Crows at dawn with all his might.

He struts around, so proud and tall,

The boldest rooster of them all!

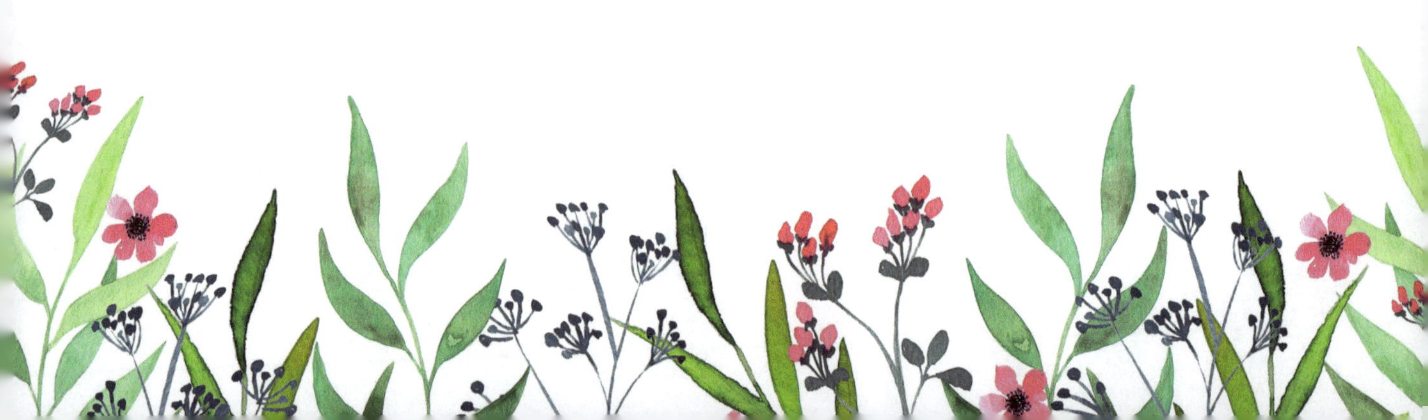

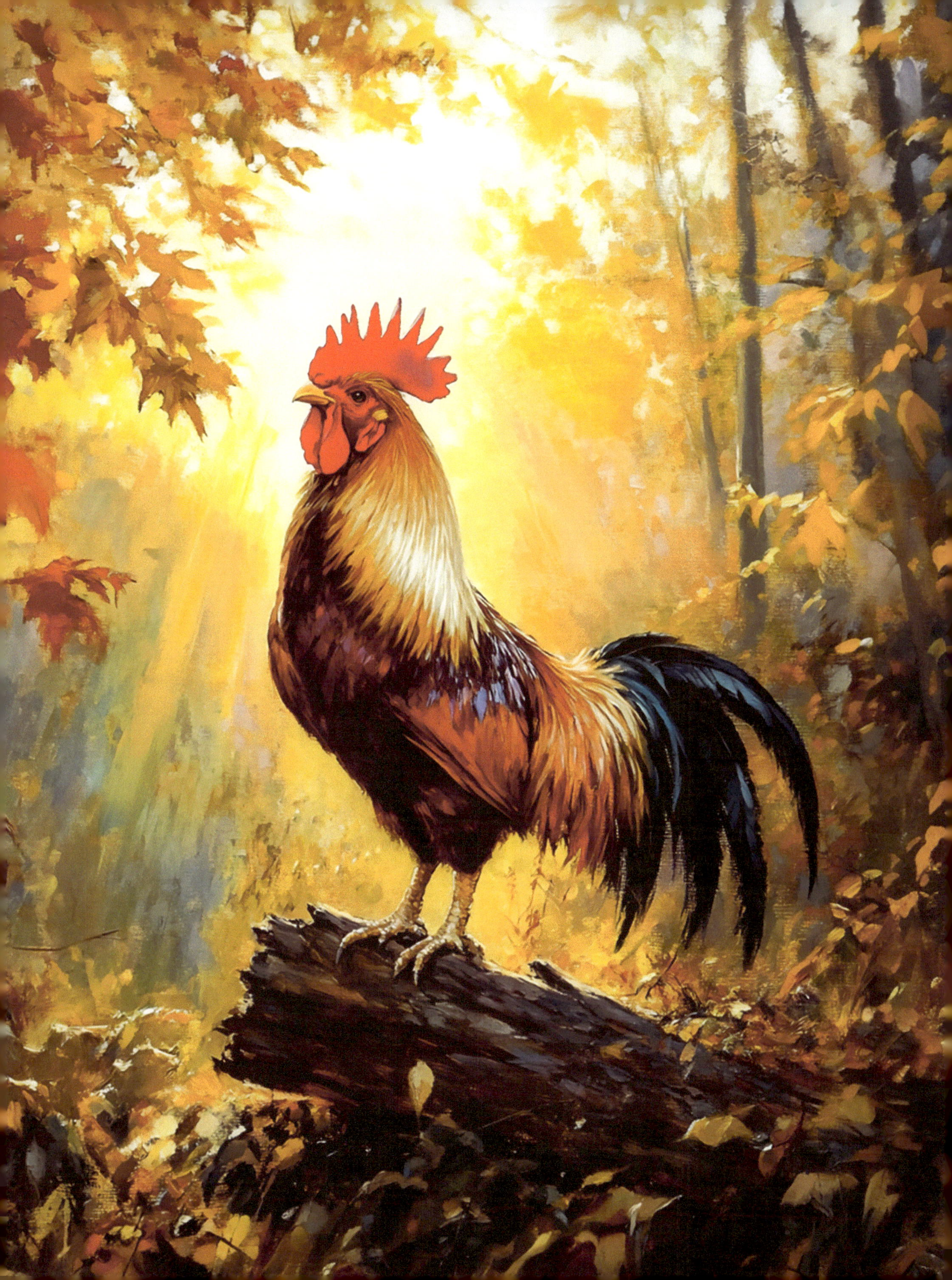

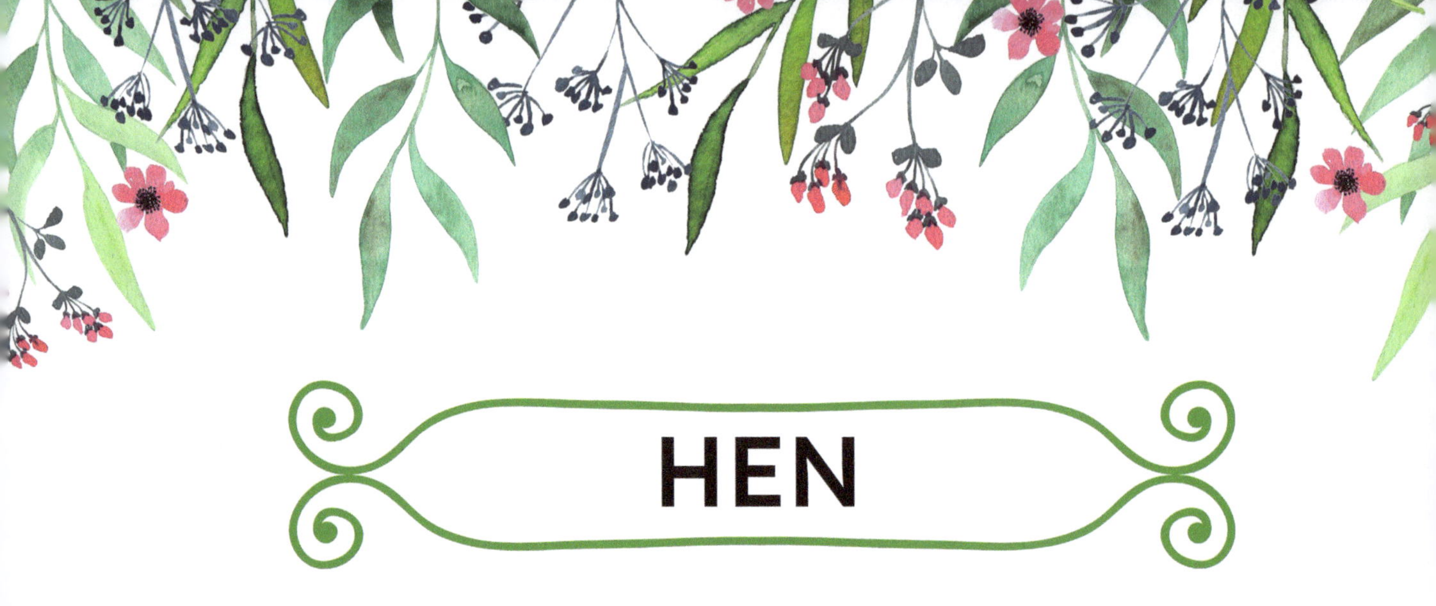

HEN

A mother hen with feathers bright,

Guides her chicks through morning light.

With gentle clucks, she leads the way,

And keeps them safe throughout the day.

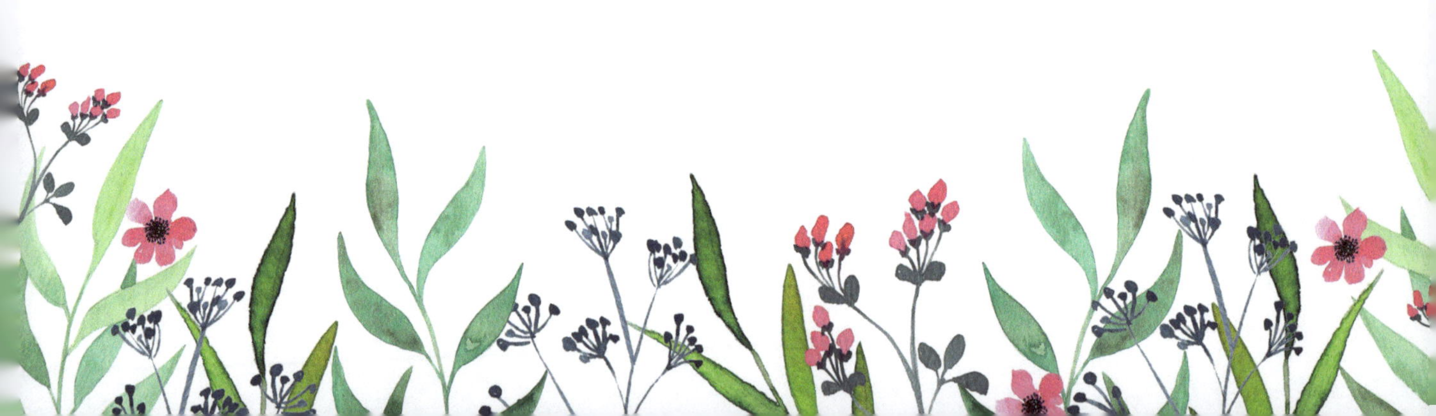

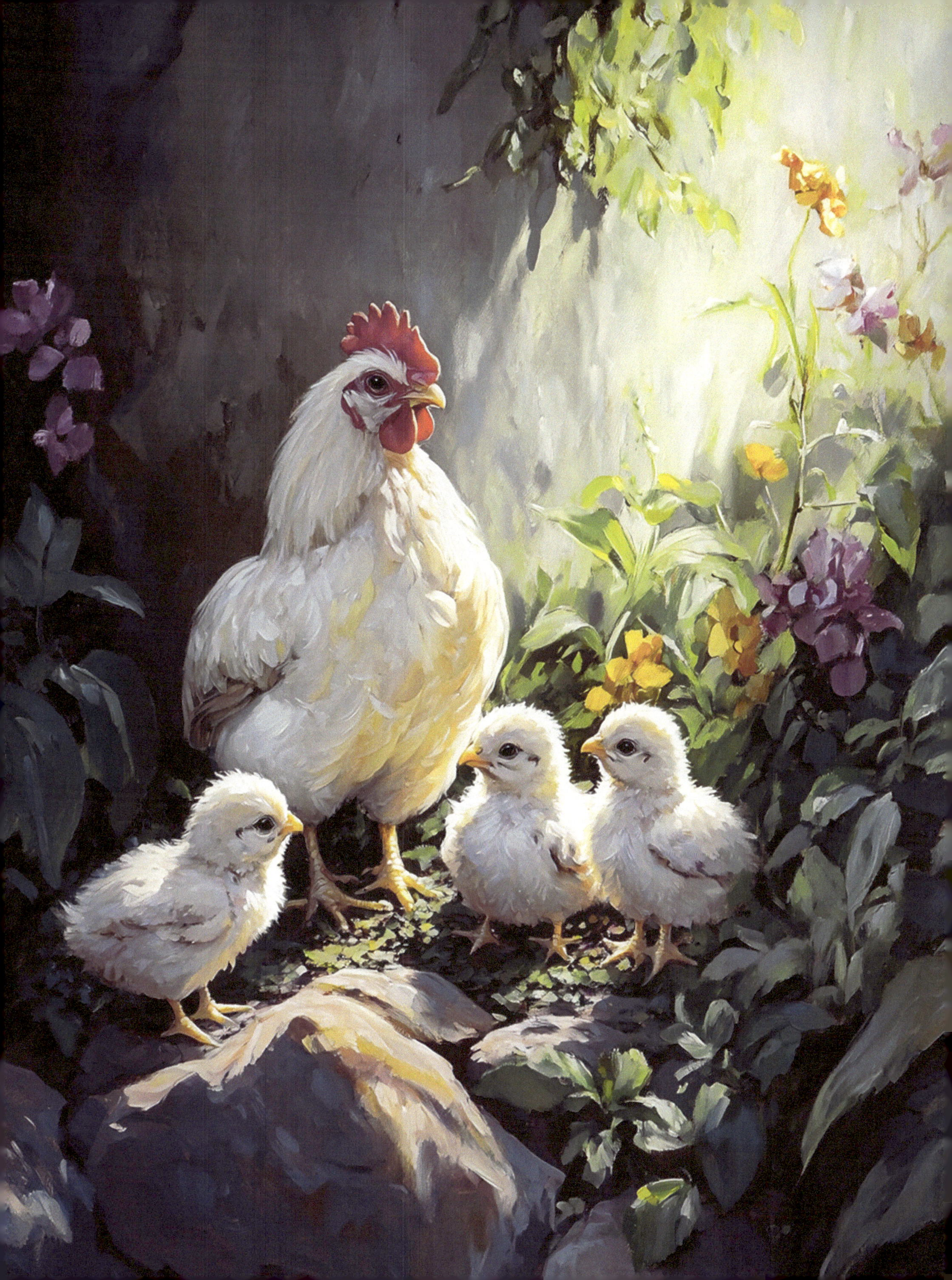

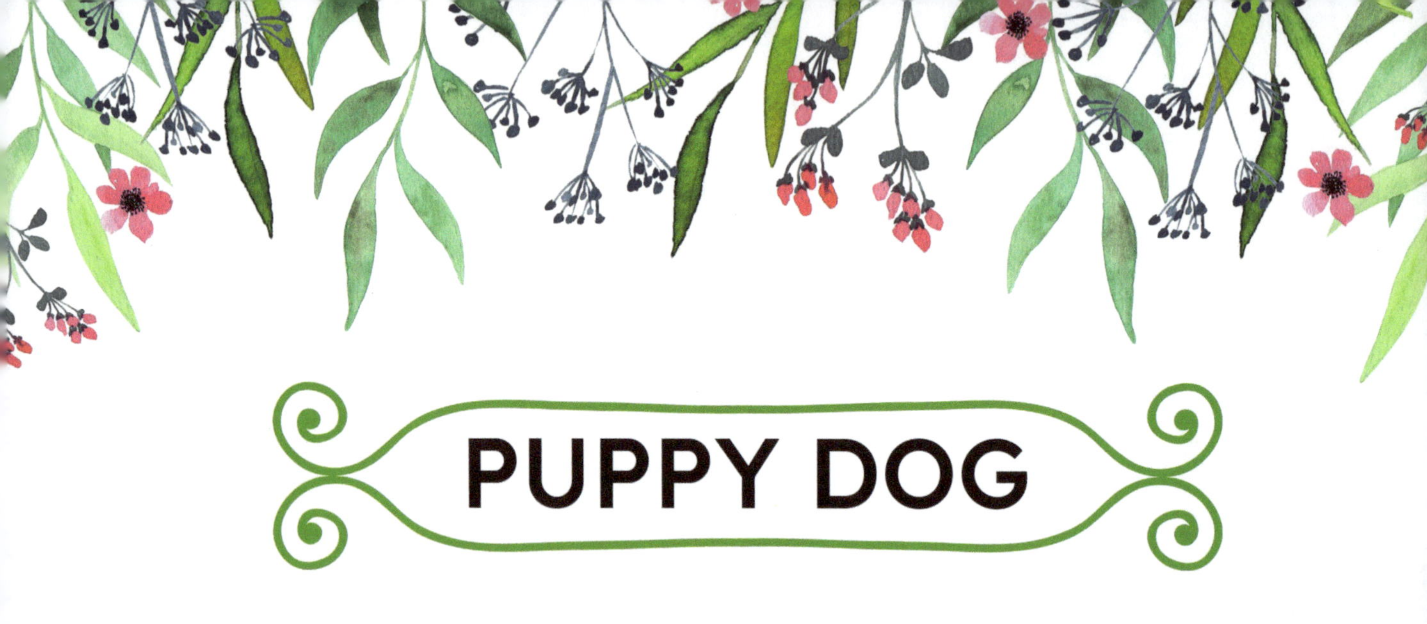

PUPPY DOG

In a garden filled with light,

Sits a puppy, golden bright.

With wagging tail and eyes alight,

He fills the world with pure delight.

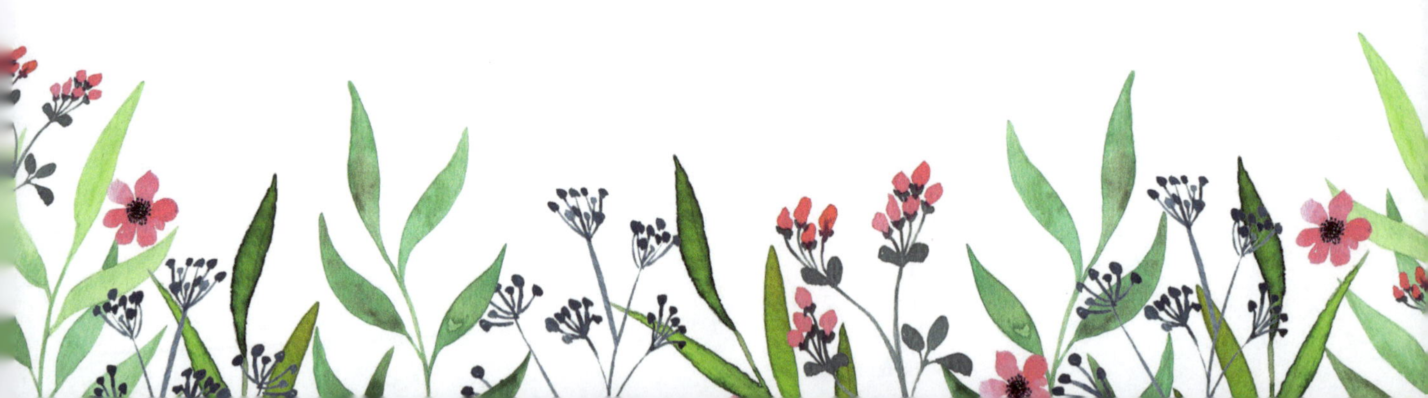

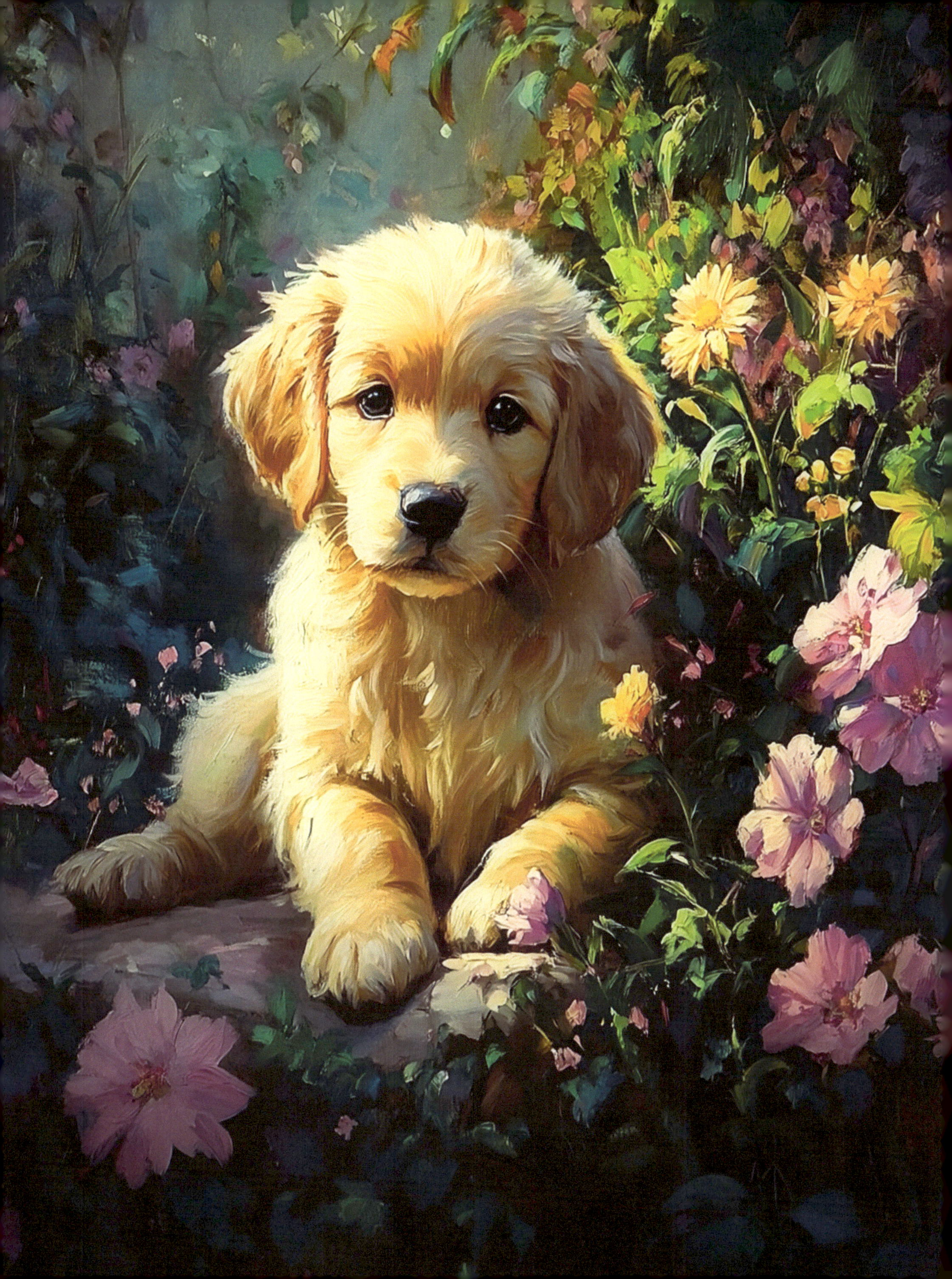

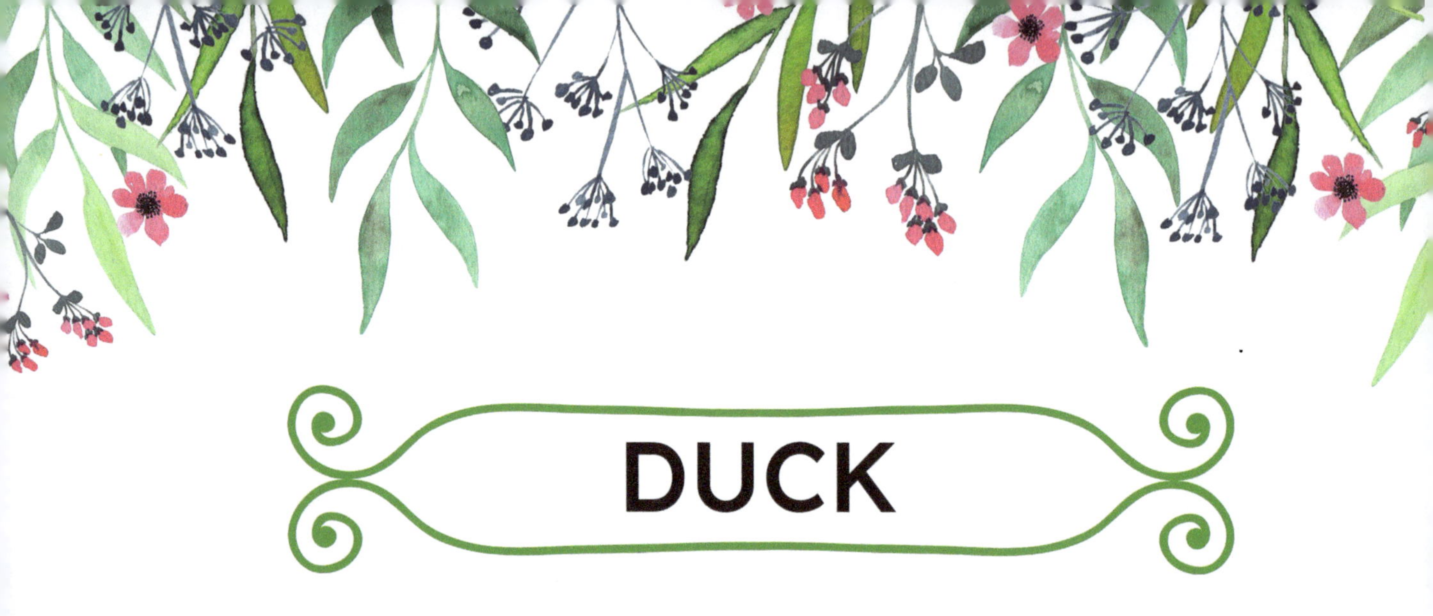

DUCK

On a pond of green and blue,

Swims a duck with ducklings new.

The ducklings paddle to and fro,

Eeny, Meeny, Miny, Moe!

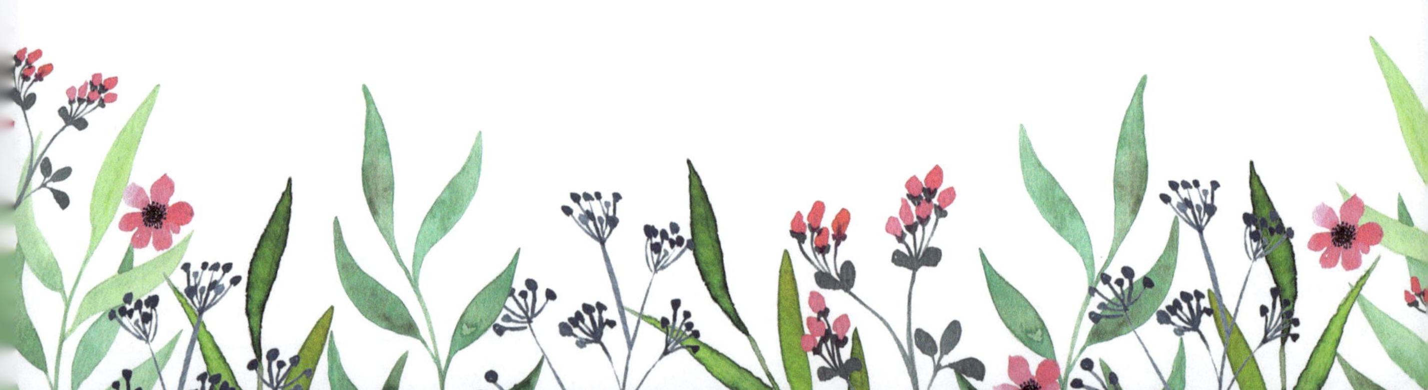

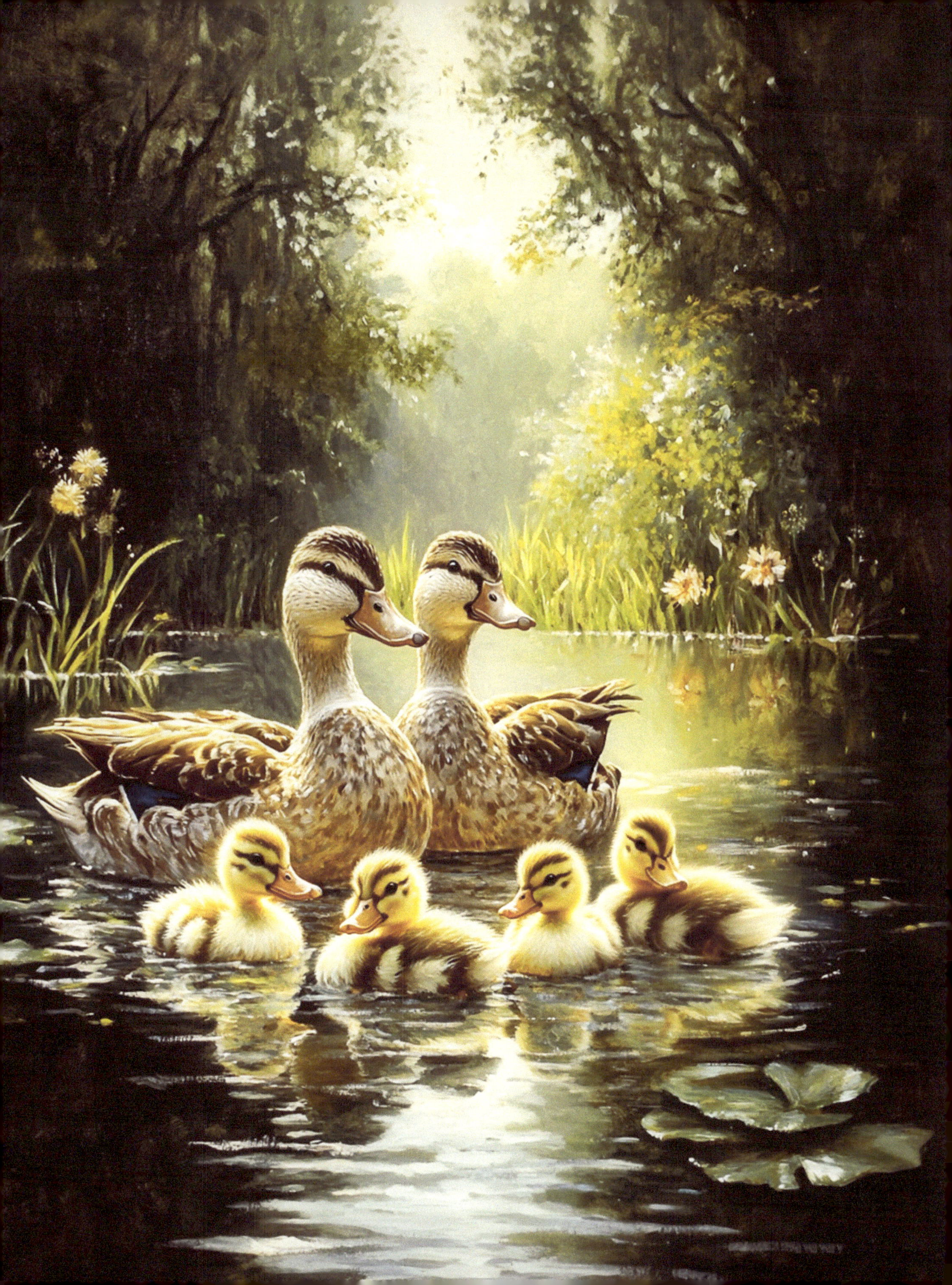

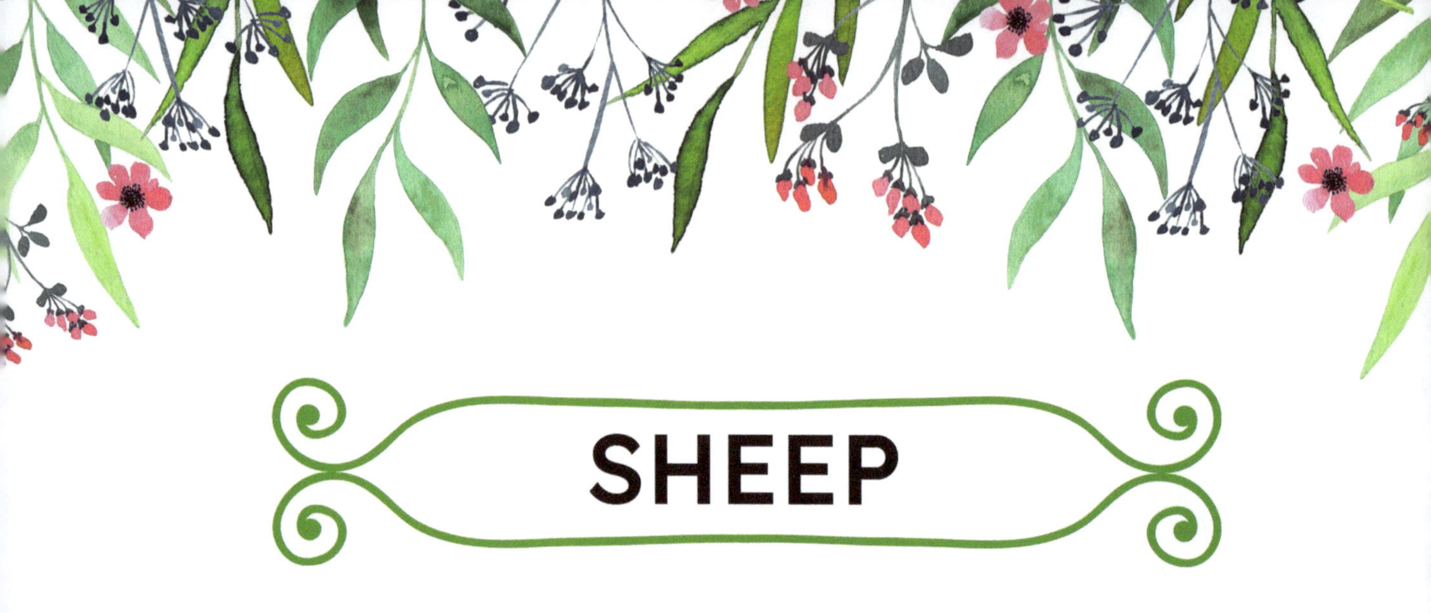

SHEEP

The hillside sheep, so fluffy and white,

Grazing in the morning light.

With gentle bleats, they roam and play,

In peaceful pastures all the day.

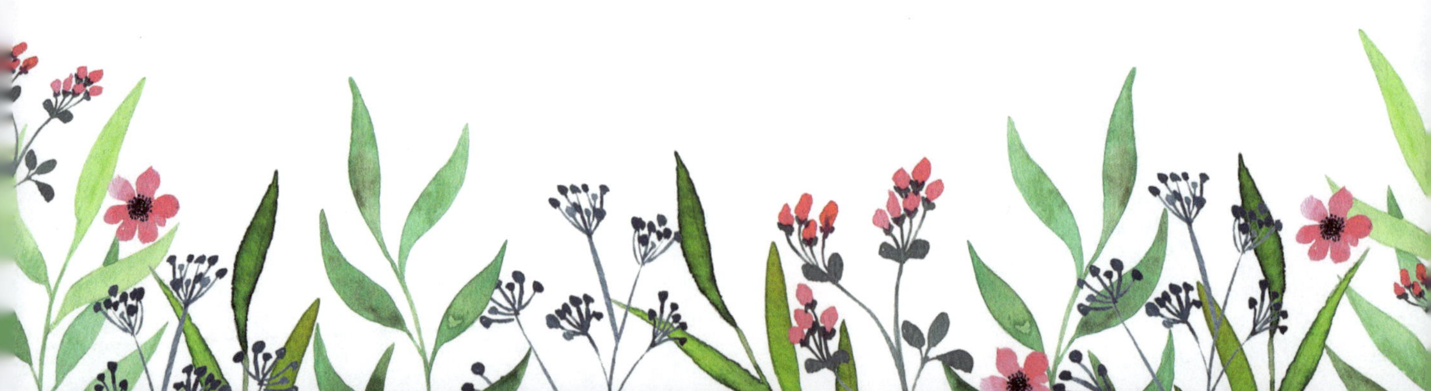

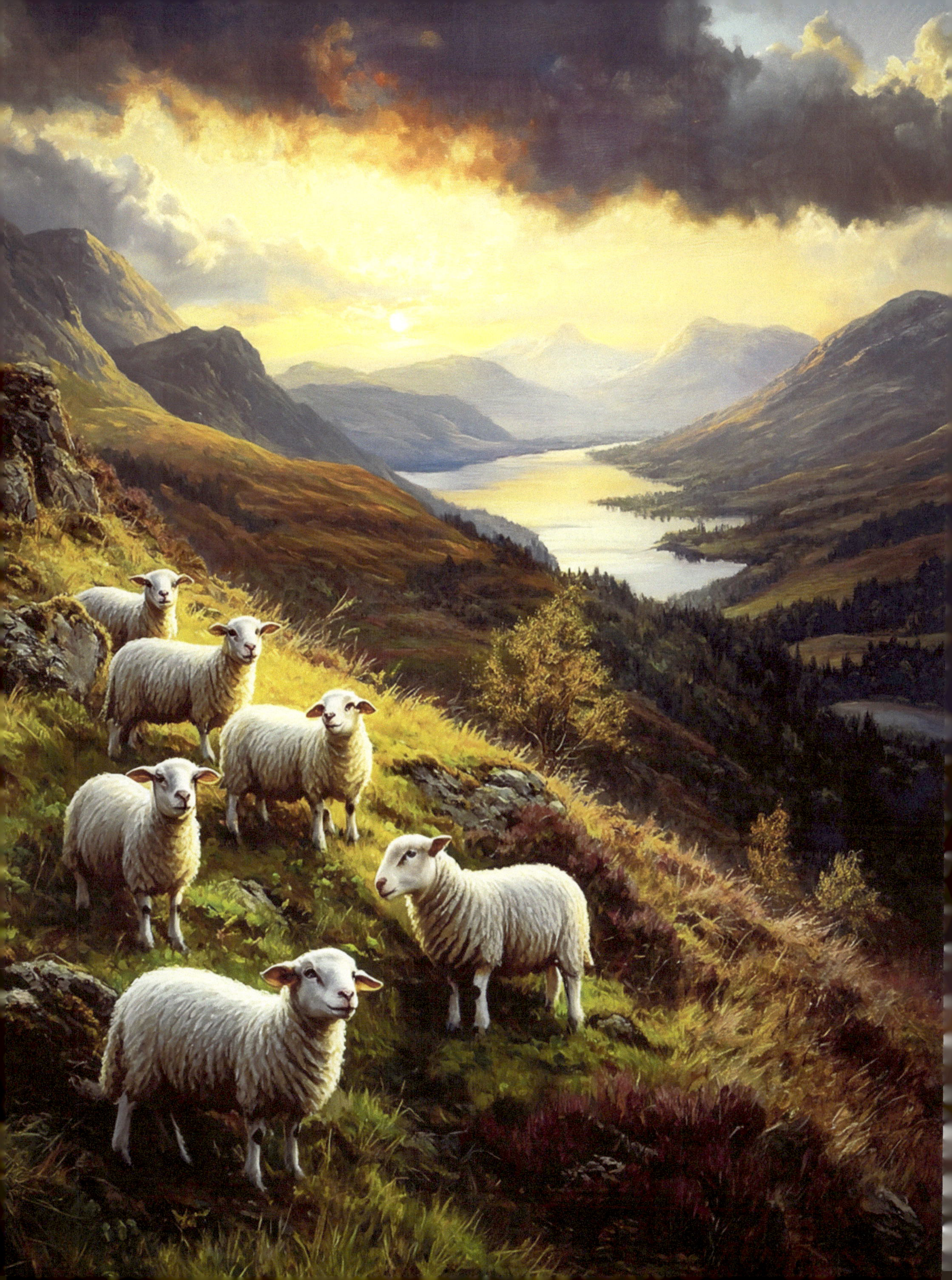

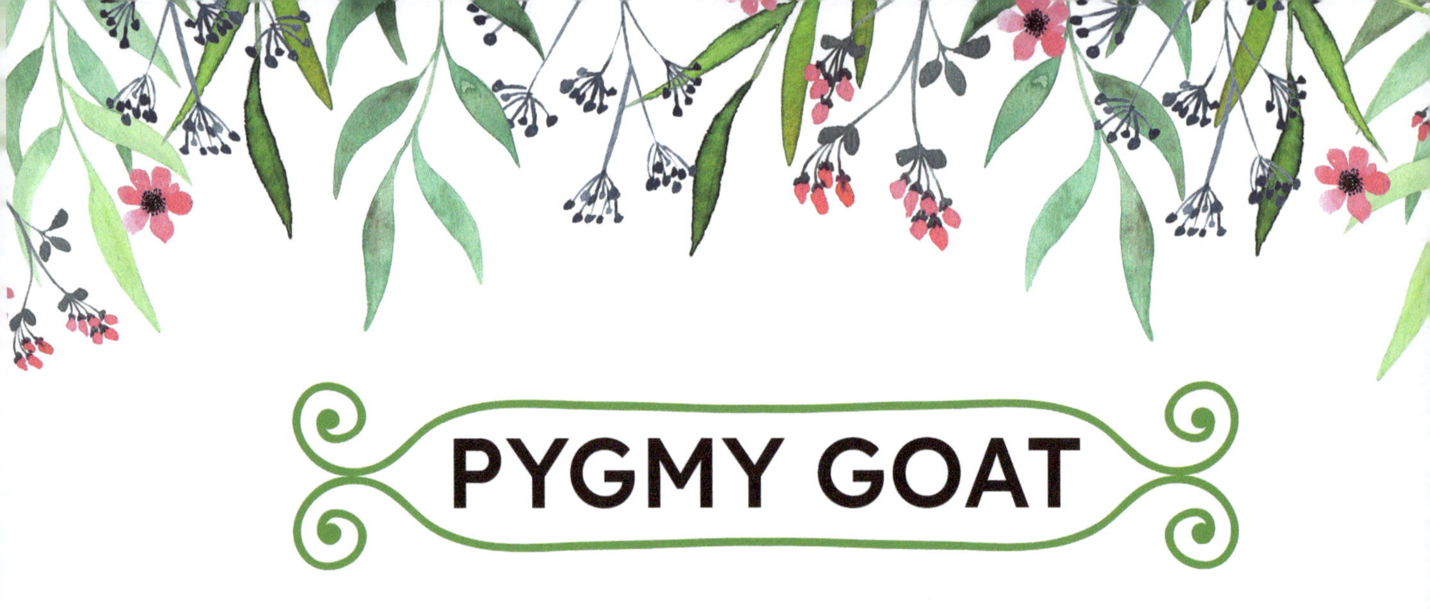

PYGMY GOAT

Goats are cheeky, goats don't care,

They eat your laundry, chew your hair.

Mischief makers, wild and free,

Climbing where they shouldn't be!

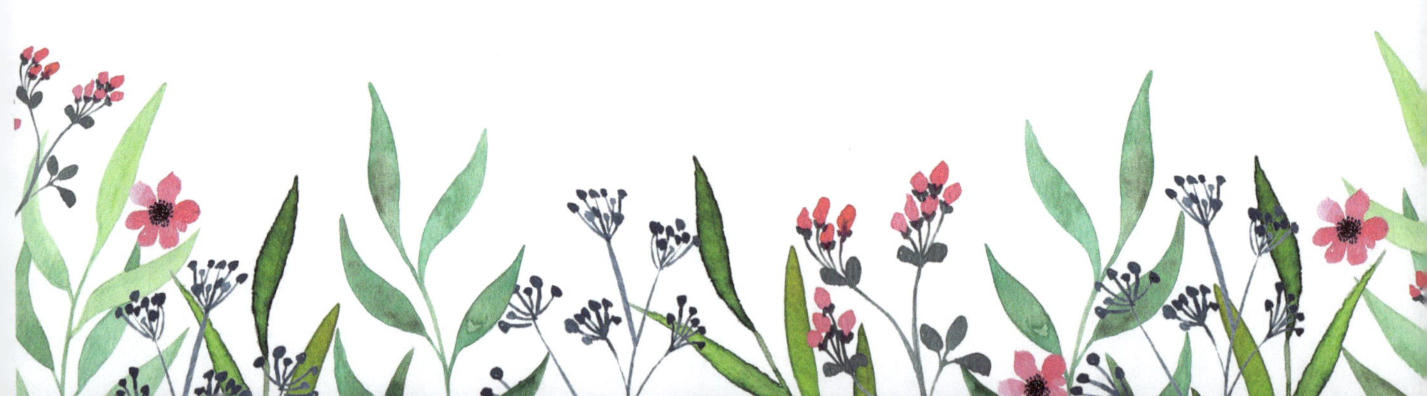

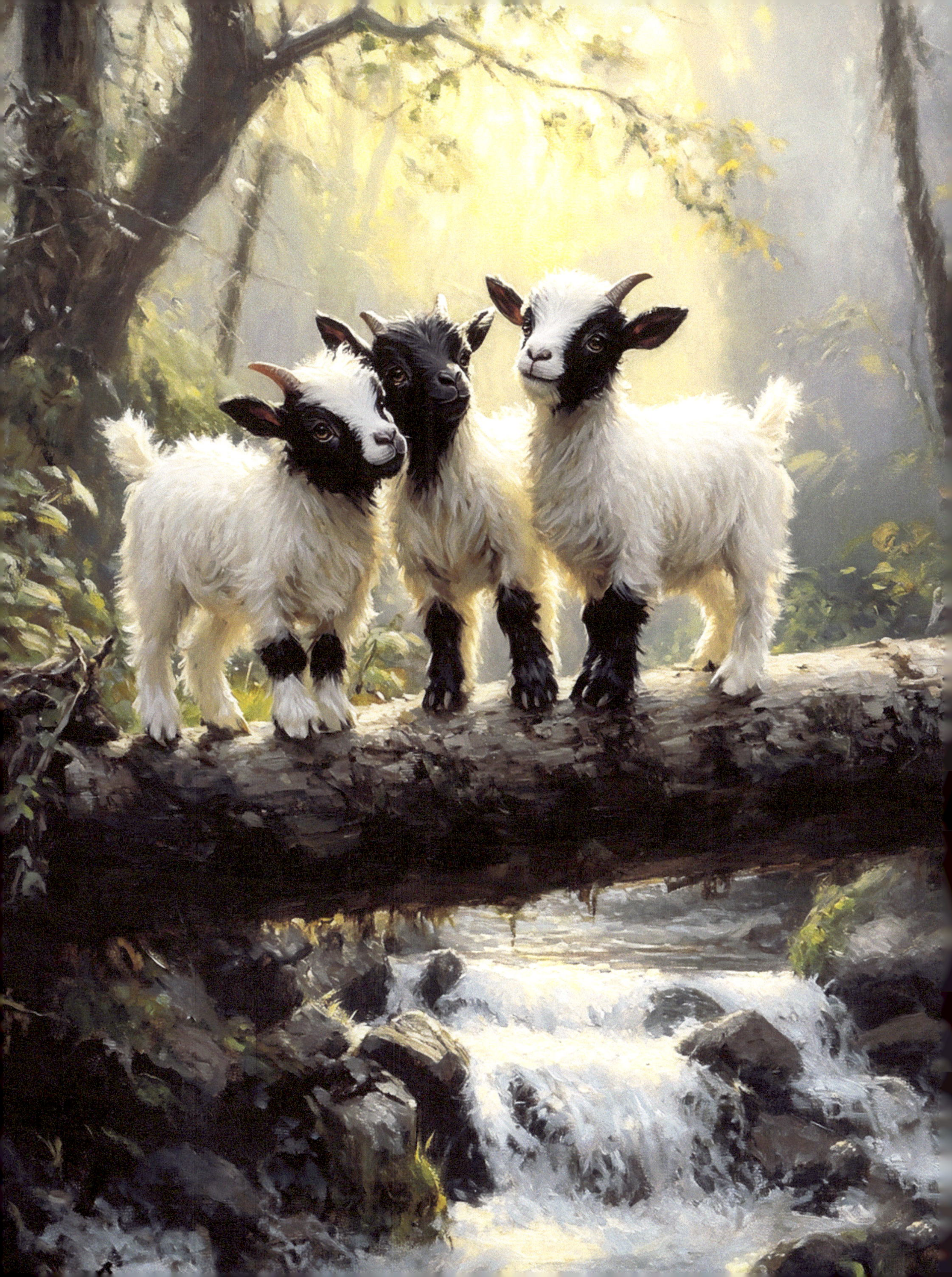

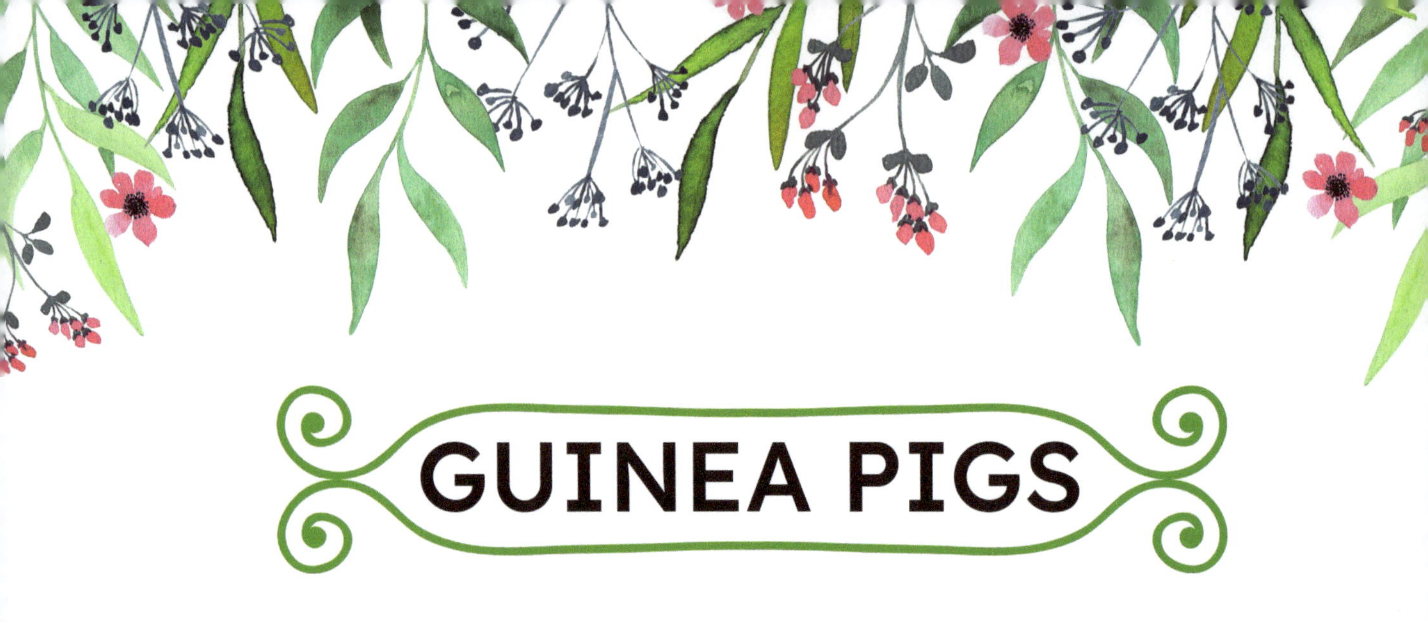

GUINEA PIGS

Guinea Pigs are lots of fun,

In fluffy lines they run and run.

They love to hide in piles of hay,

But their chubby sides give them away.

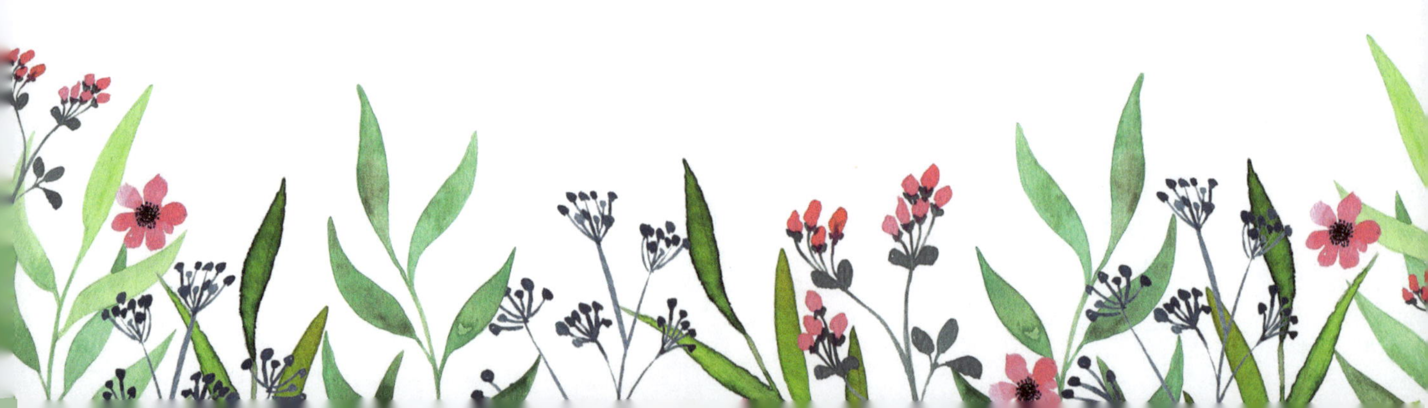

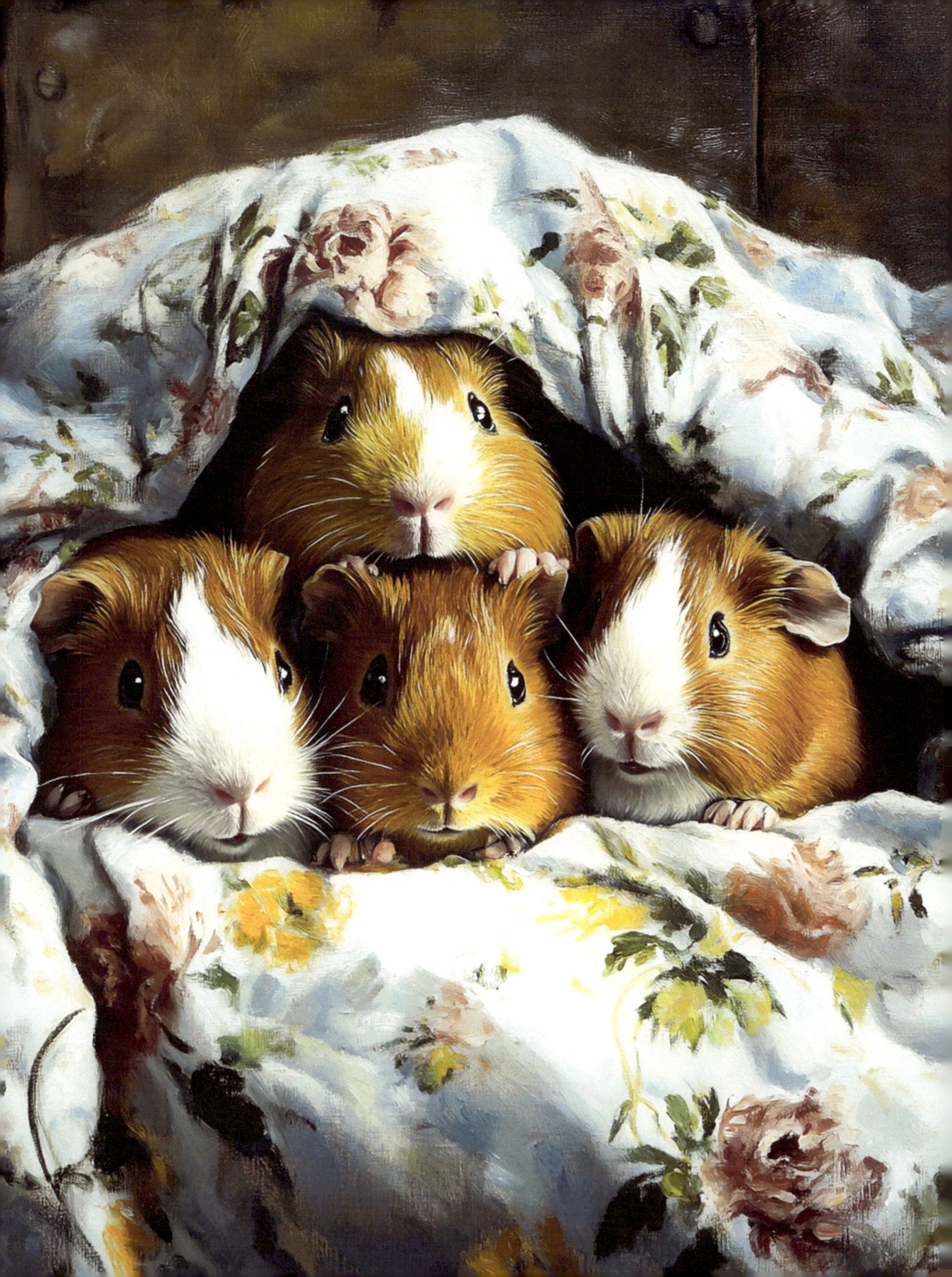

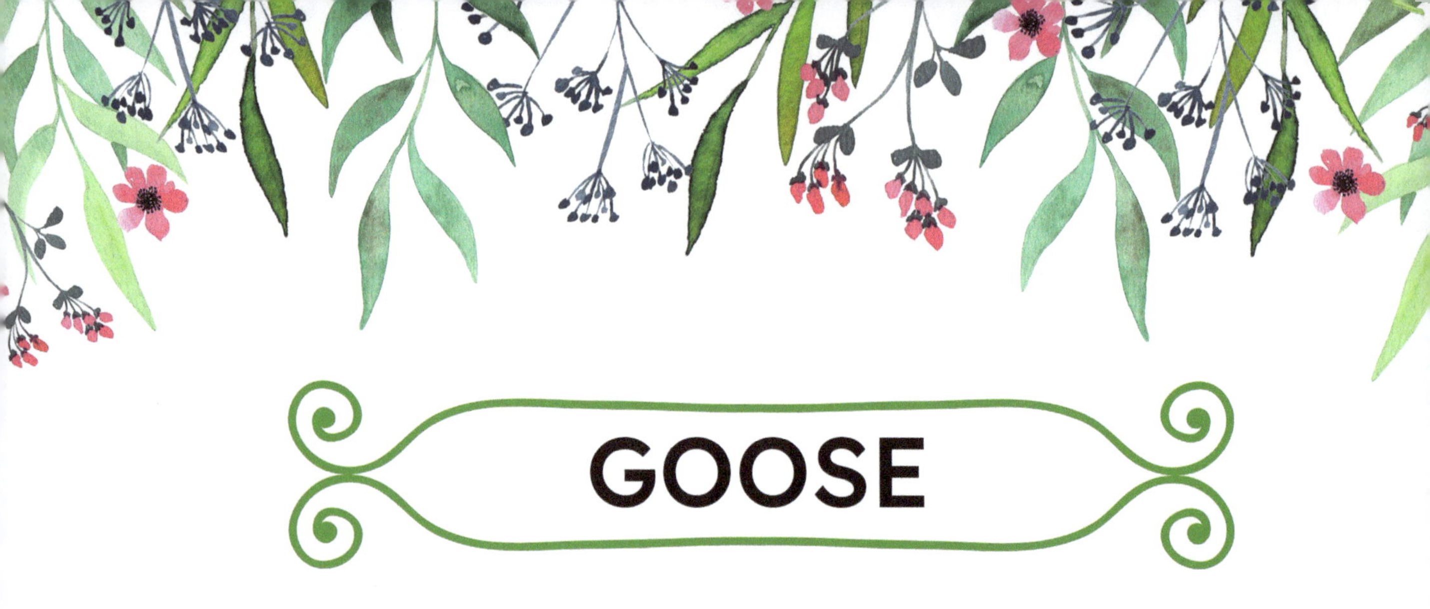

GOOSE

A fluffy goose with feathers white,

Waddles round in morning light.

She honks hello with happy cheer,

A friendly face that's always near.

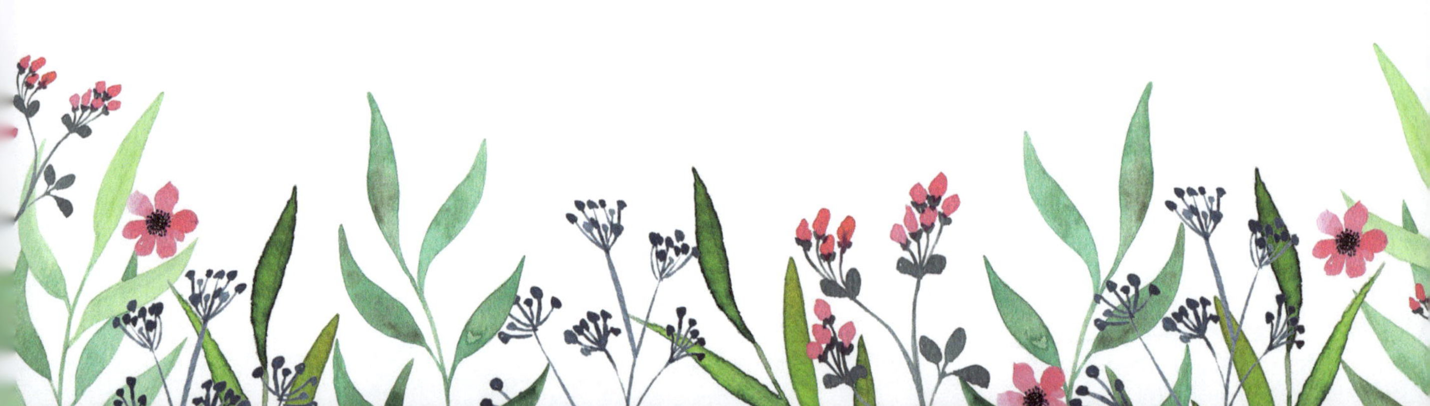

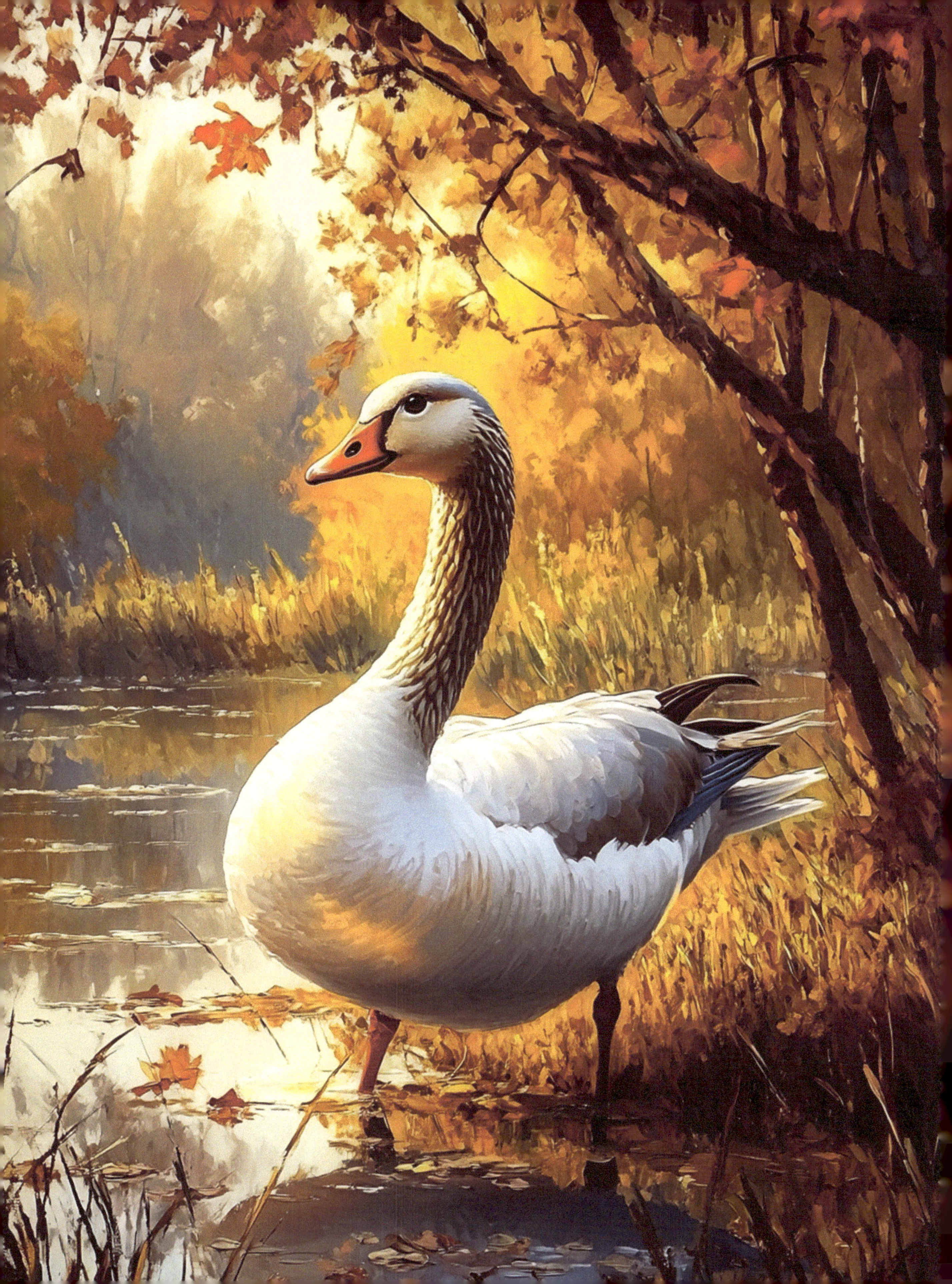

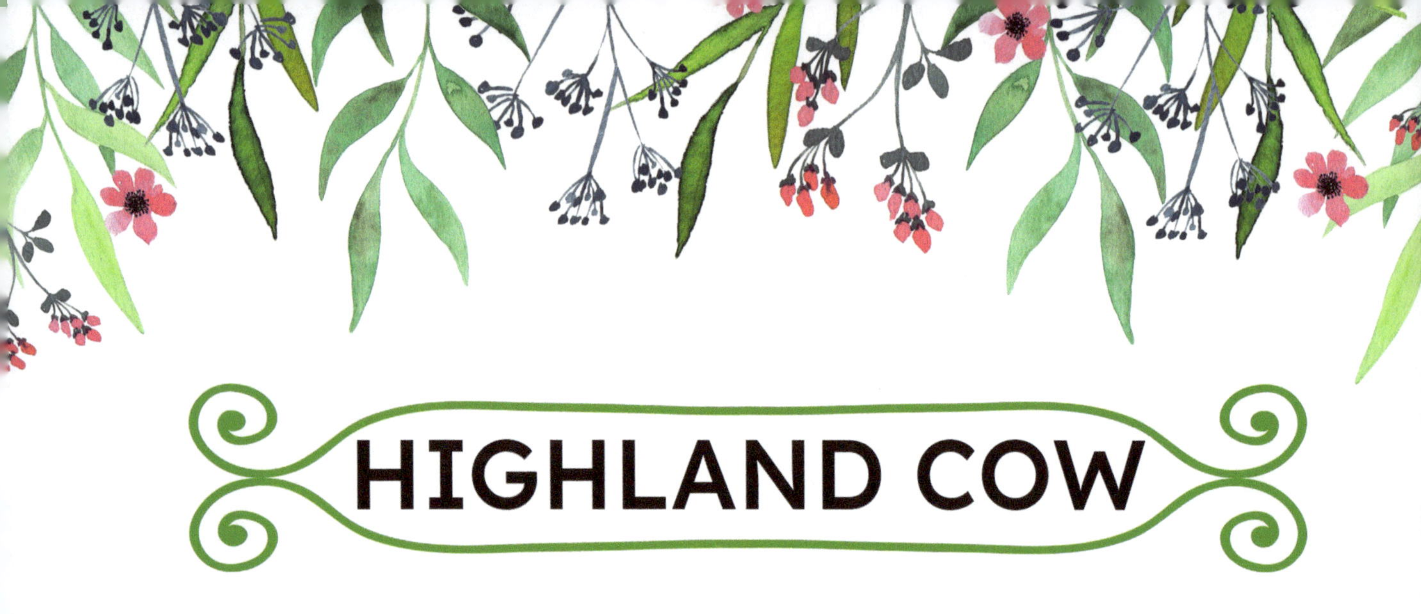

HIGHLAND COW

A Scottish cow with coat so long,

Gentle eyes and horns so strong.

She thinks her hair's the latest style,

A walking wig that makes you smile!

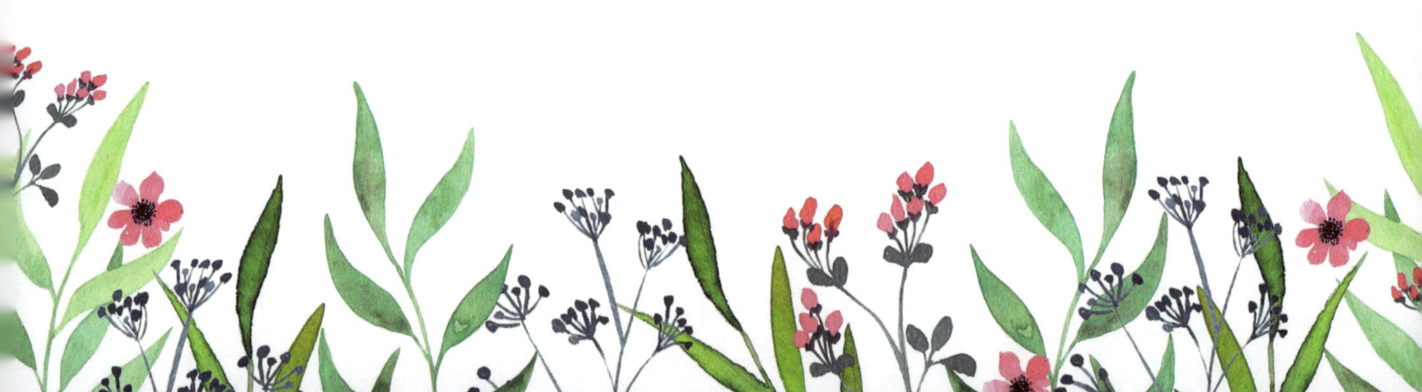

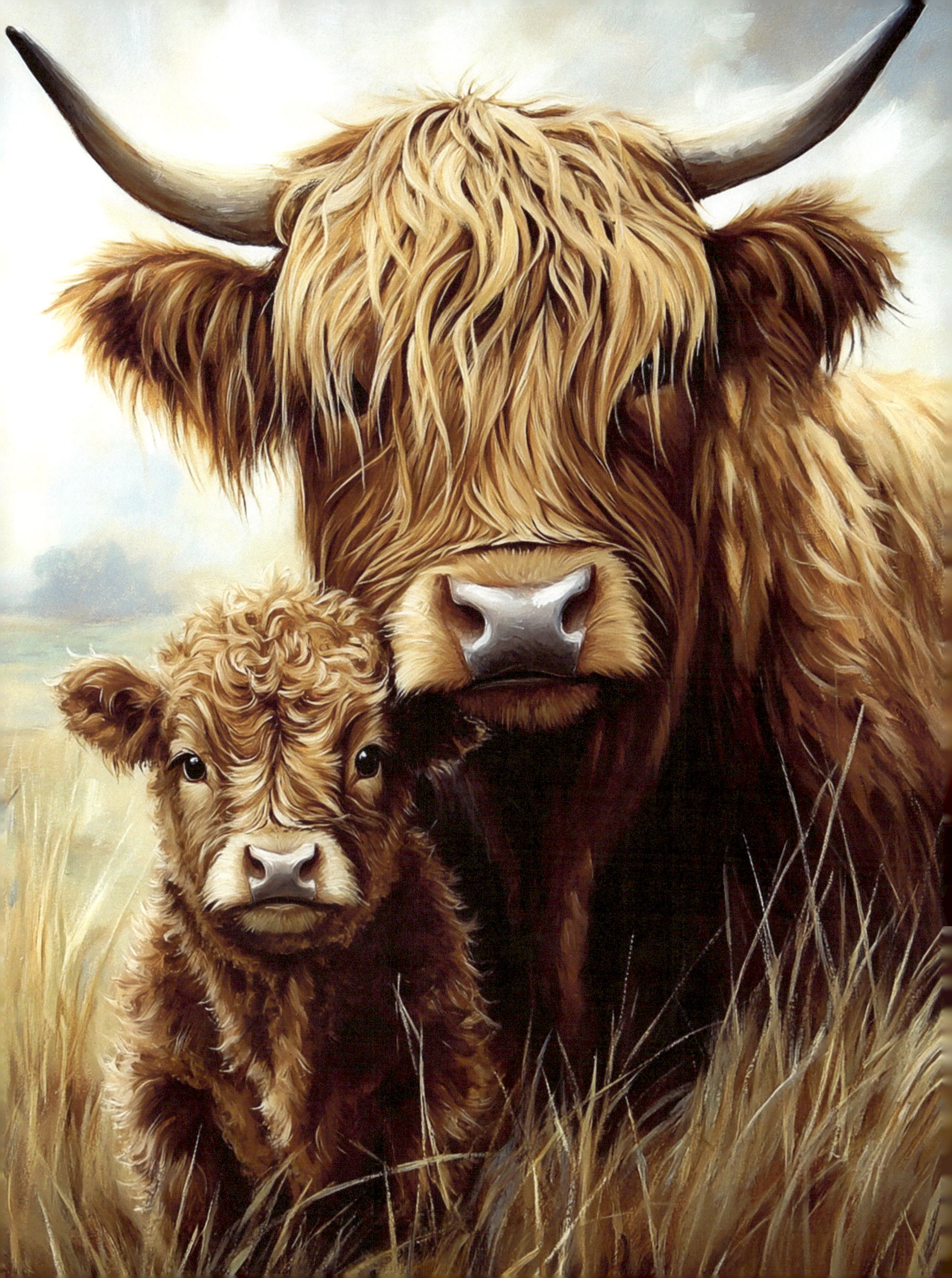

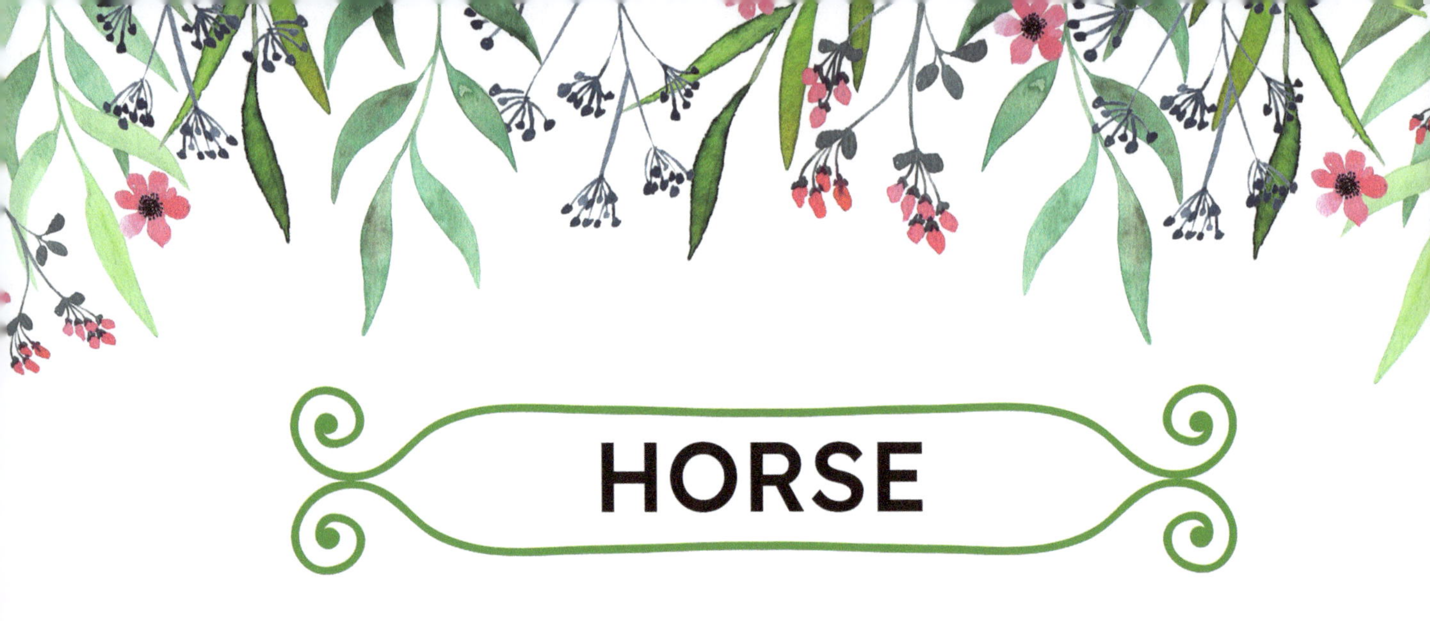

HORSE

Majestic mane and flowing tail,

Galloping free 'cross hill and dale.

Strength and grace in every stride,

A noble spirit, wild and wise.

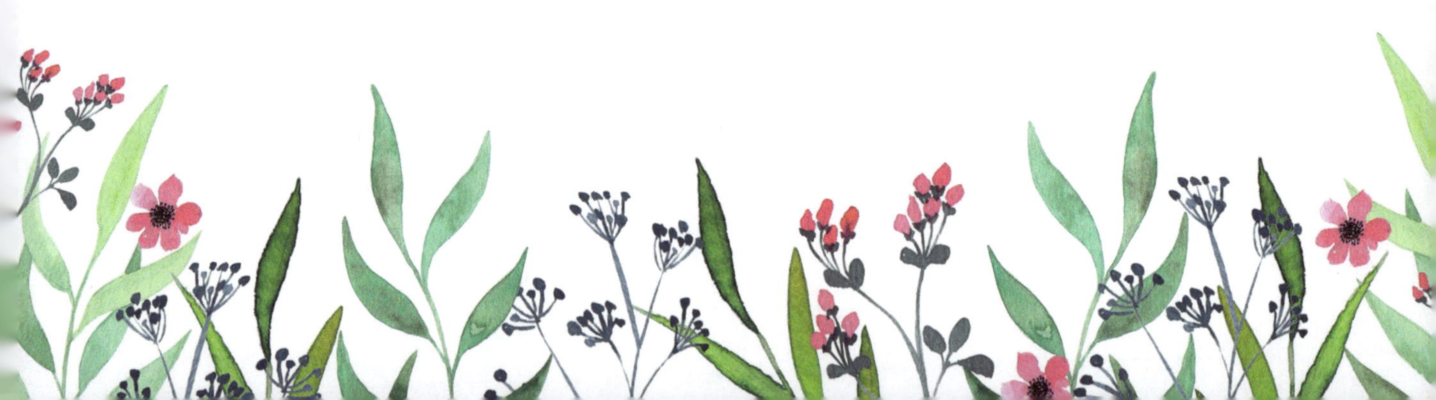

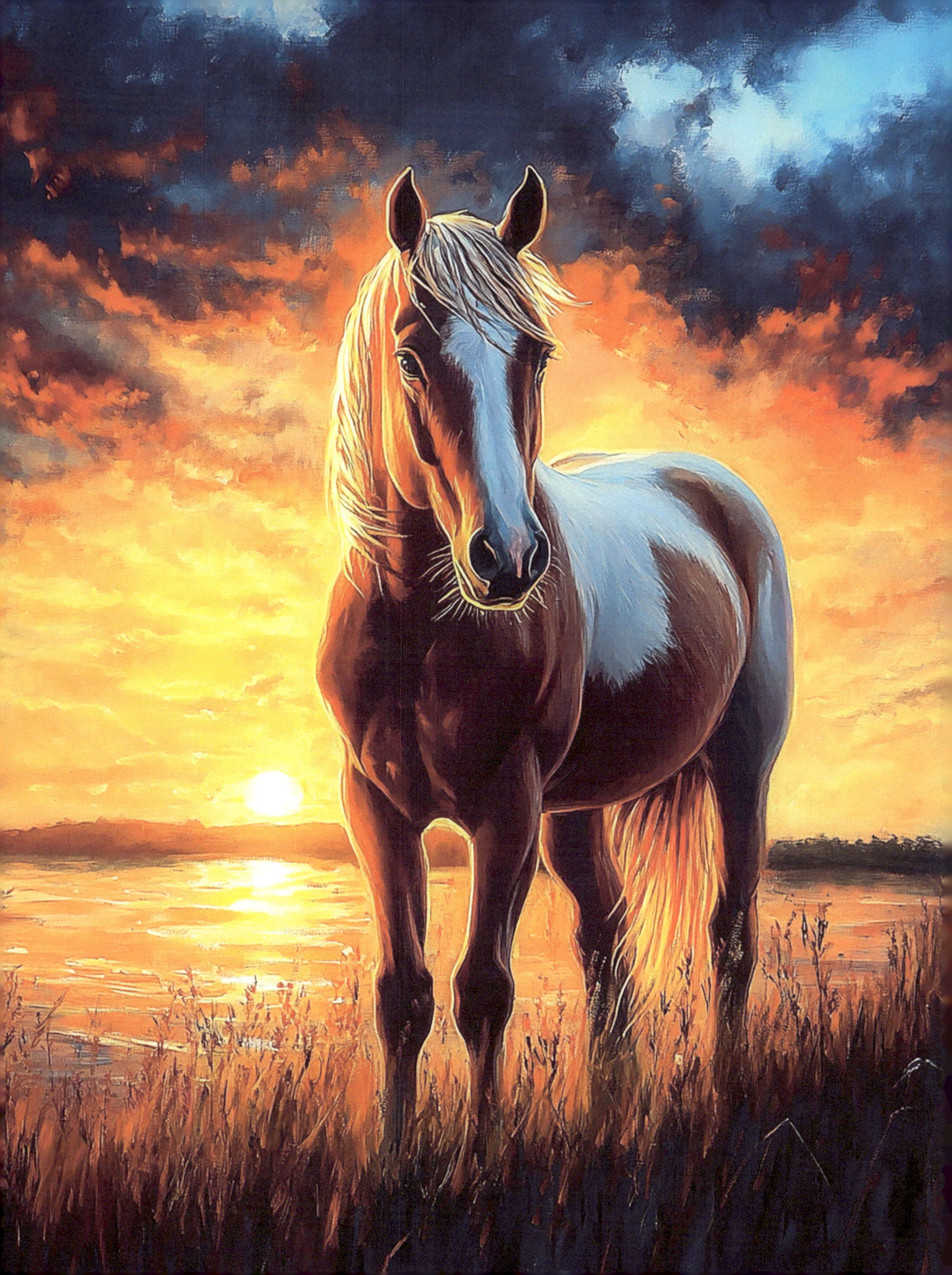

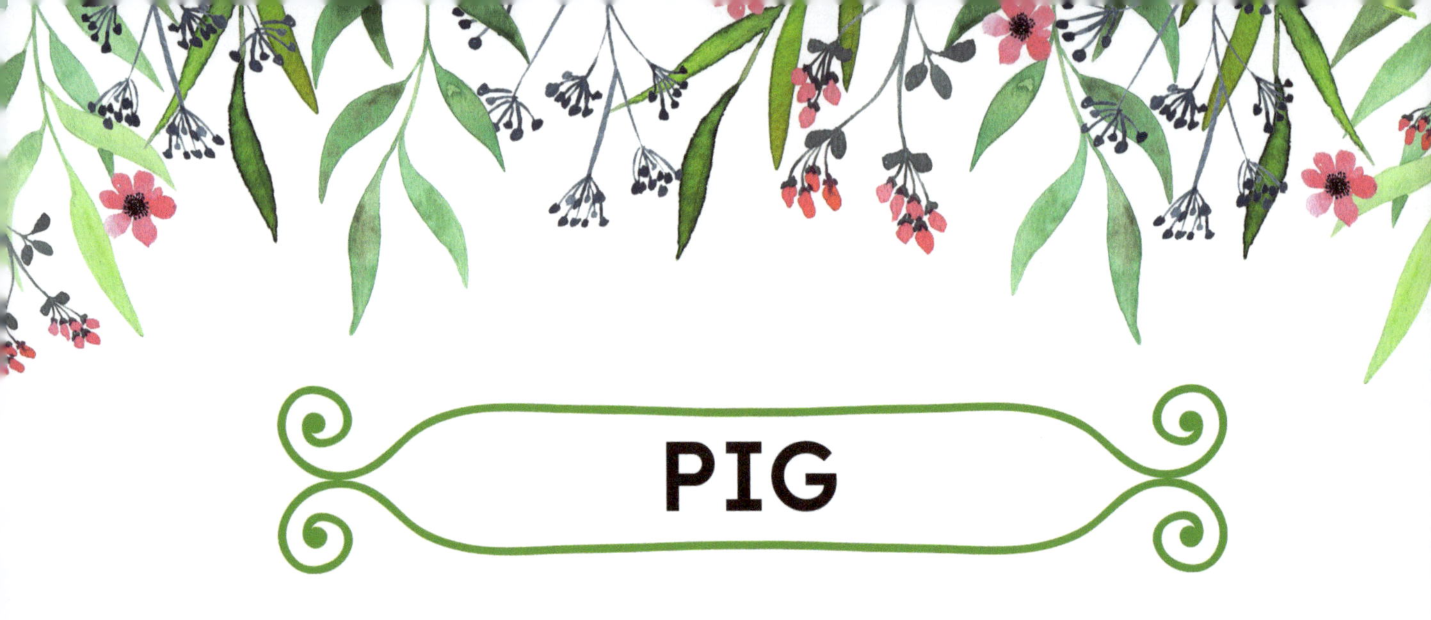

PIG

The pig is clever, he's no fool,

He rolls in mud to keep his cool.

Friendly, playful, cute and fun,

The piggy loves to swim and run.

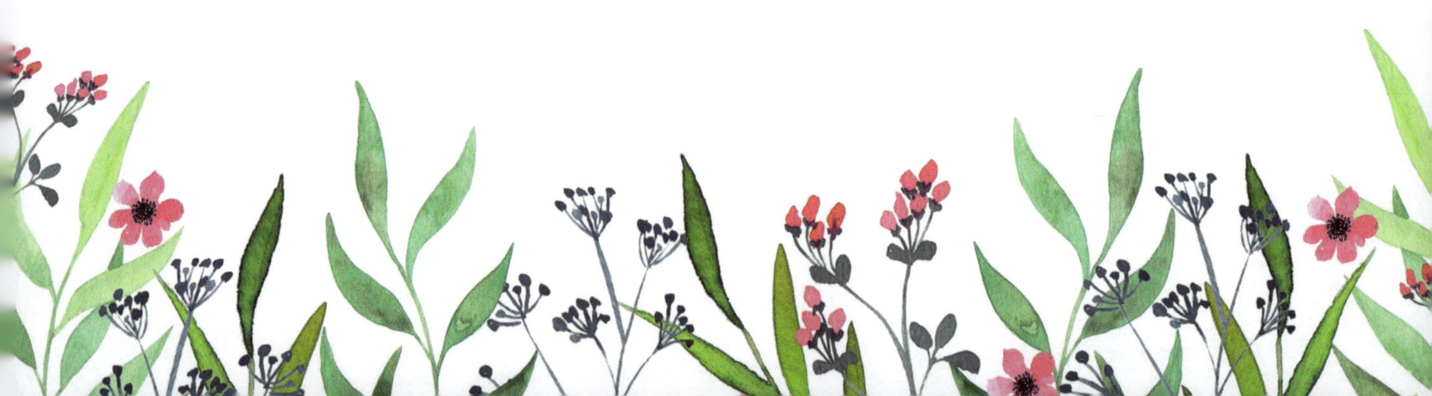

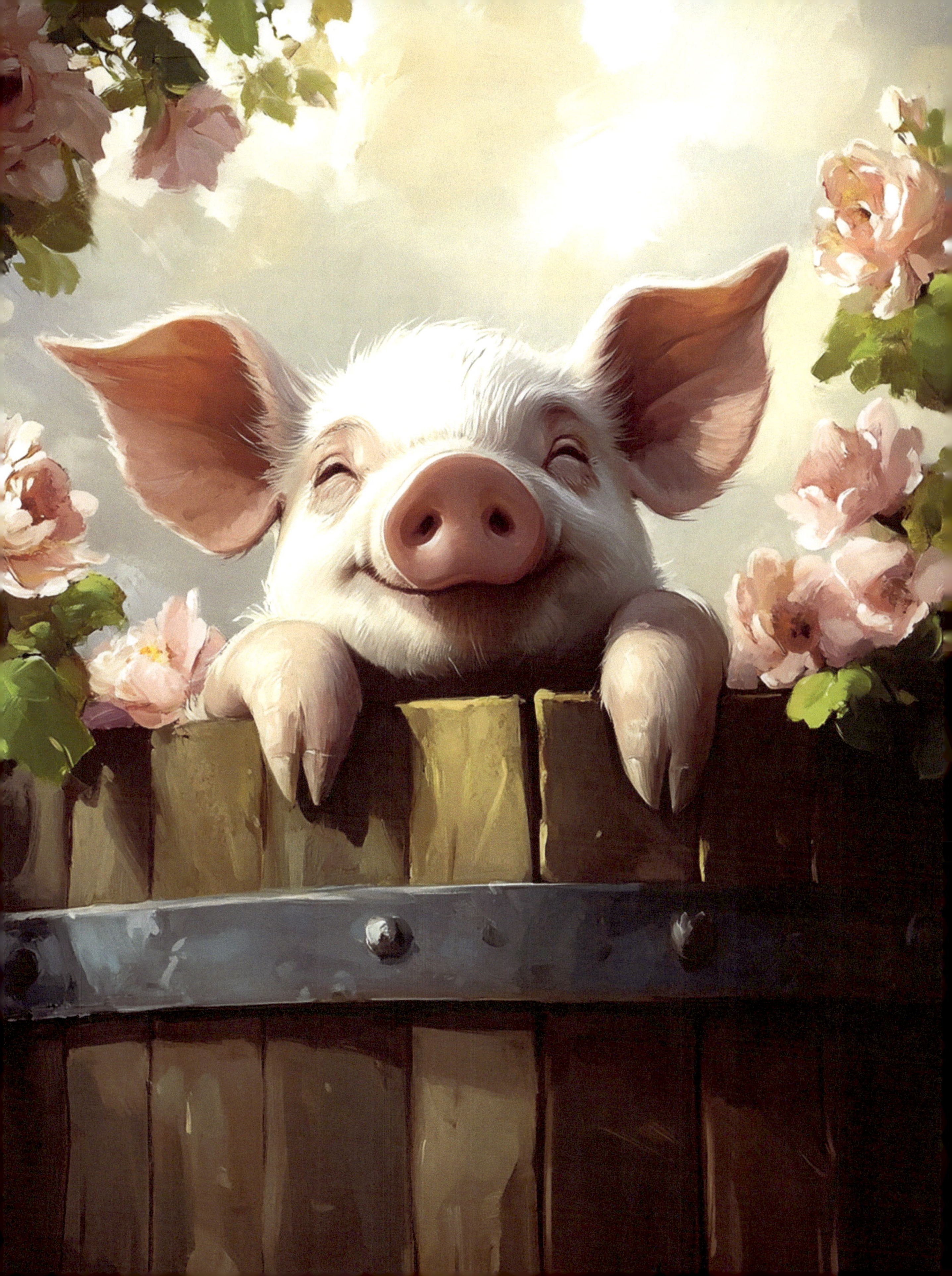

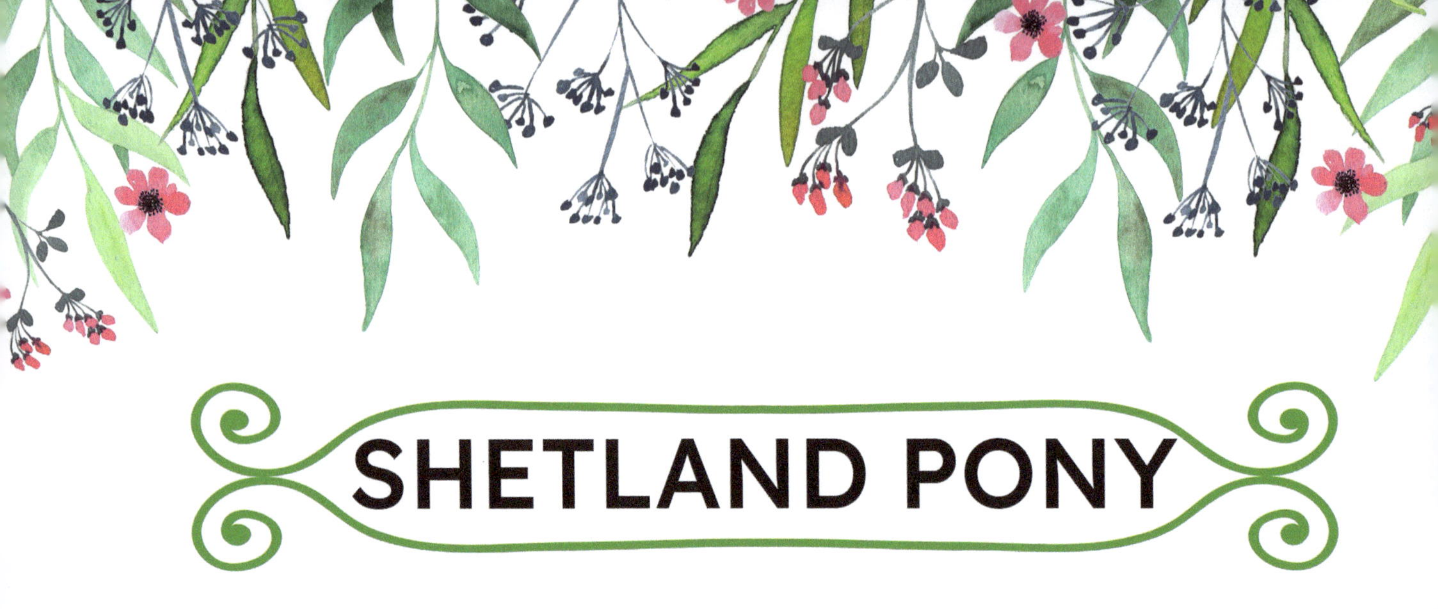

SHETLAND PONY

A Shetland pony, small and sweet,

Has tiny hooves and prancing feet.

With twinkling eyes and mane so bright,

A tiny horse that's pure delight!

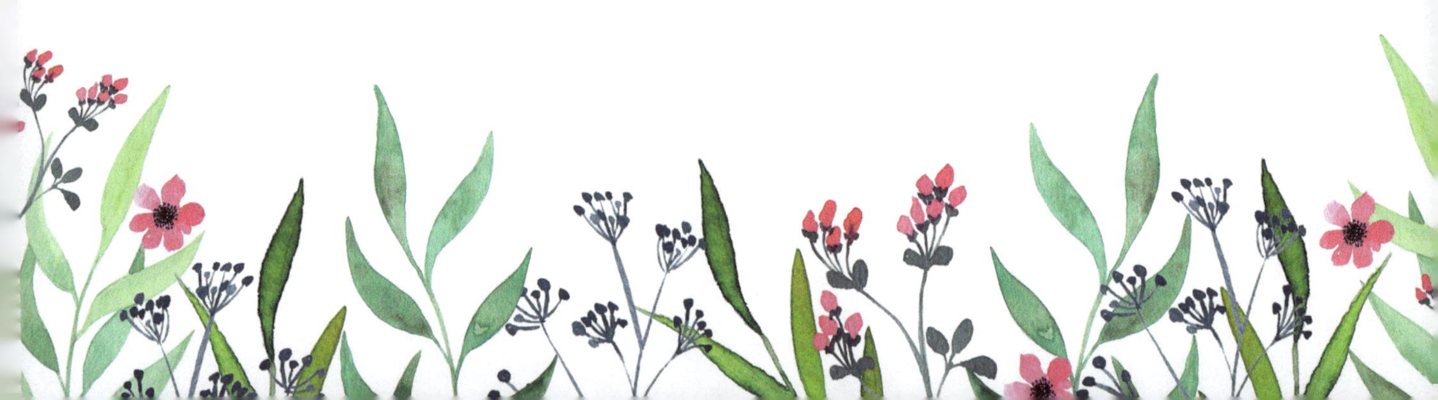

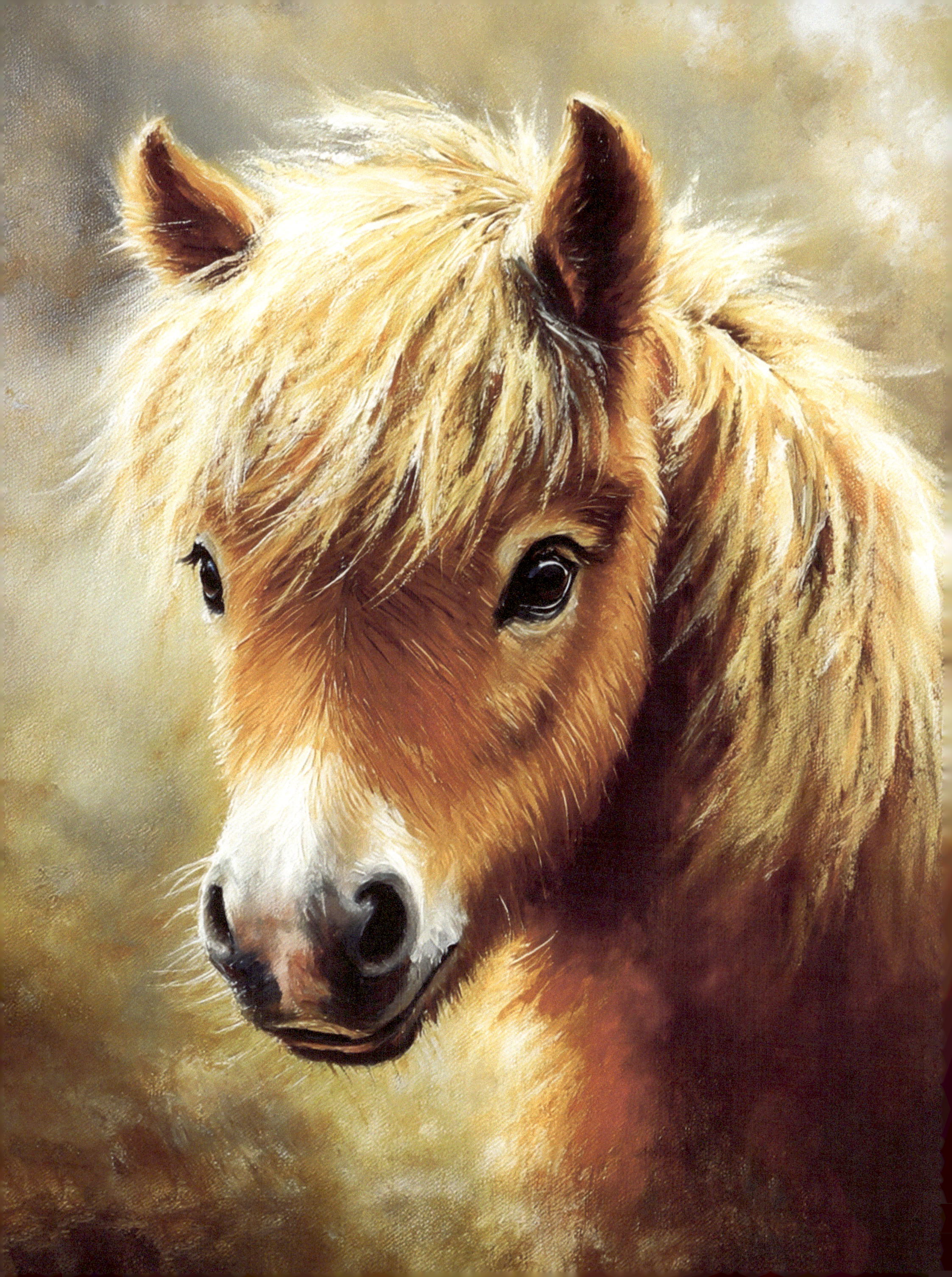

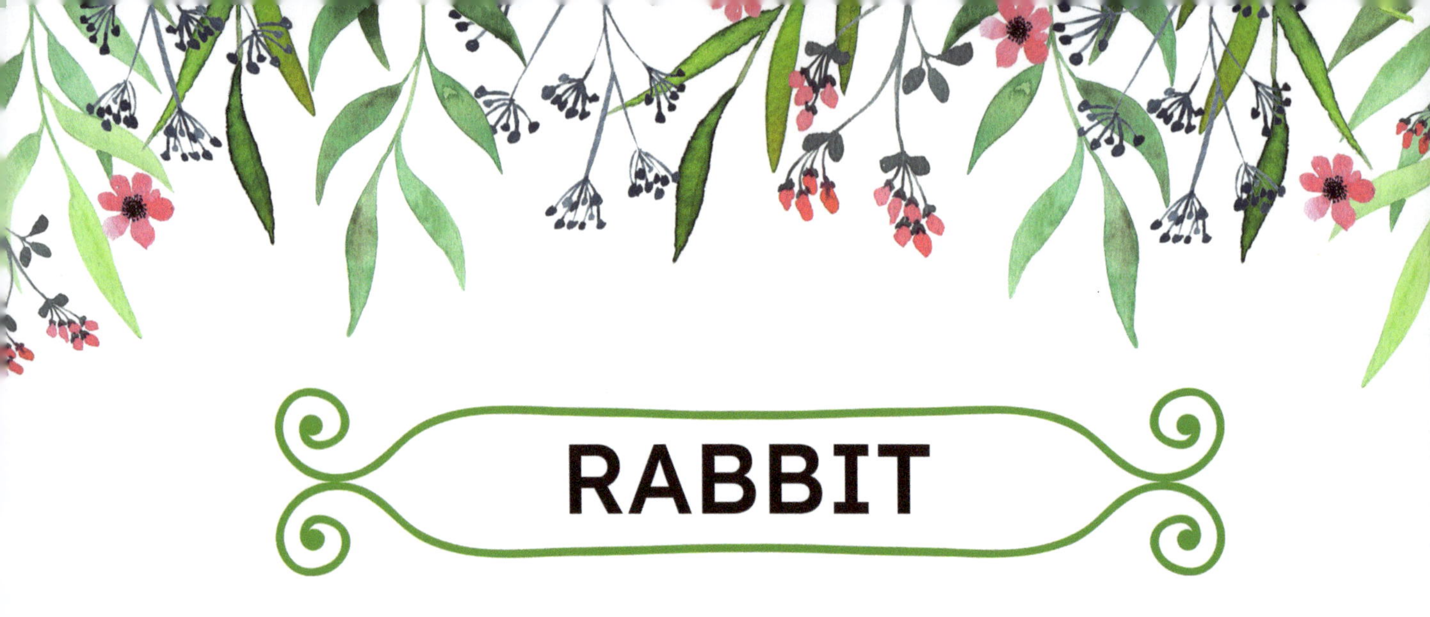

RABBIT

Mother rabbit, soft and kind,

Two sweet bunnies right behind.

Fluffy tails and twitching nose,

Off they hop where clover grows.

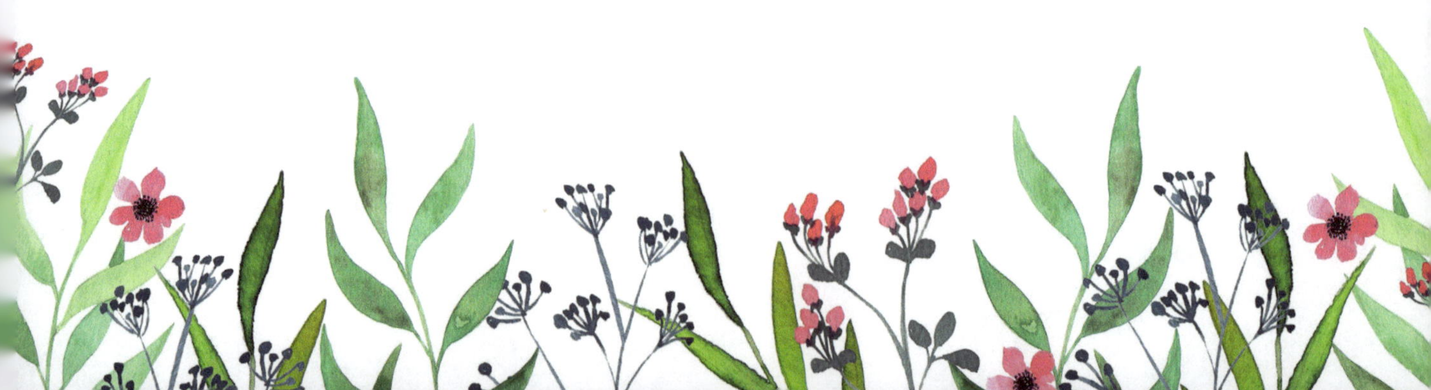

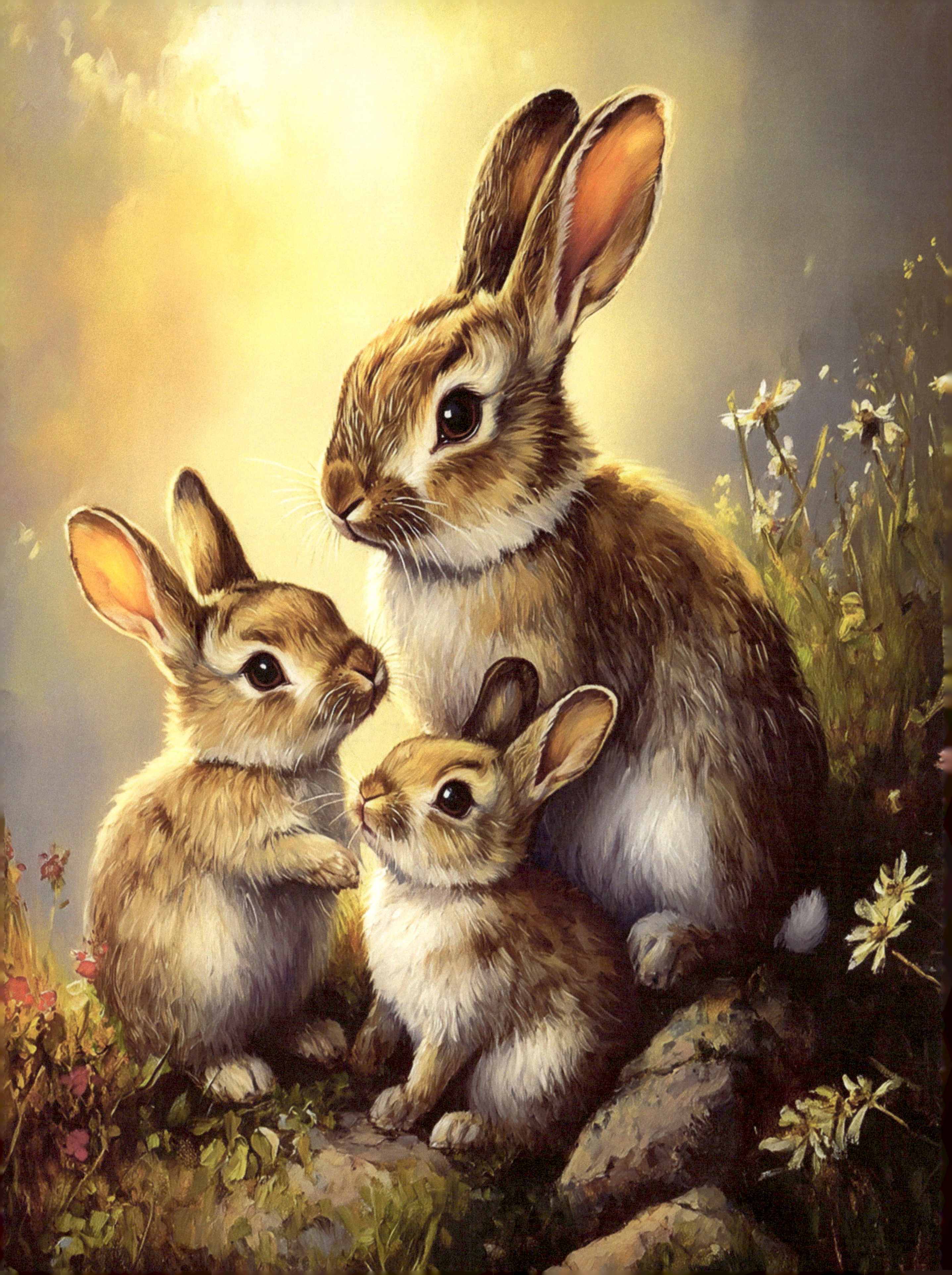

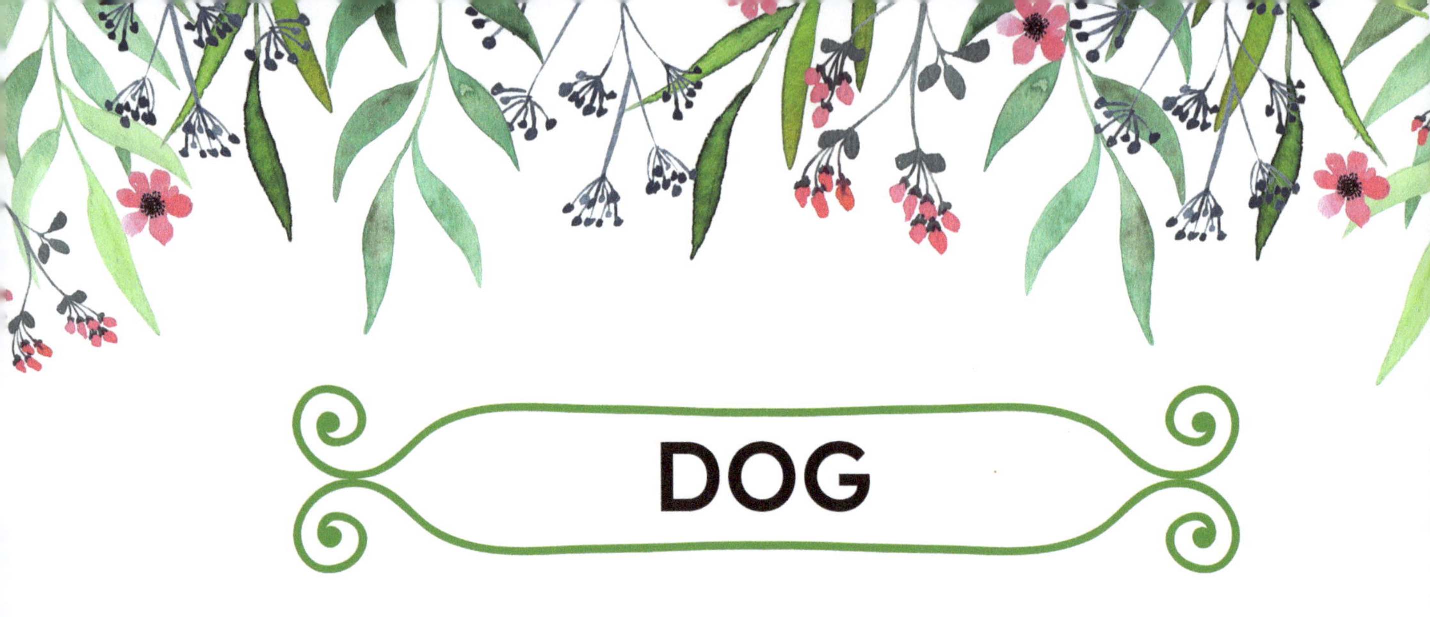

DOG

A loyal dog with heart so true,

In every step, stays close to you.

With gentle eyes and loving paw,

The sweetest love you ever saw.

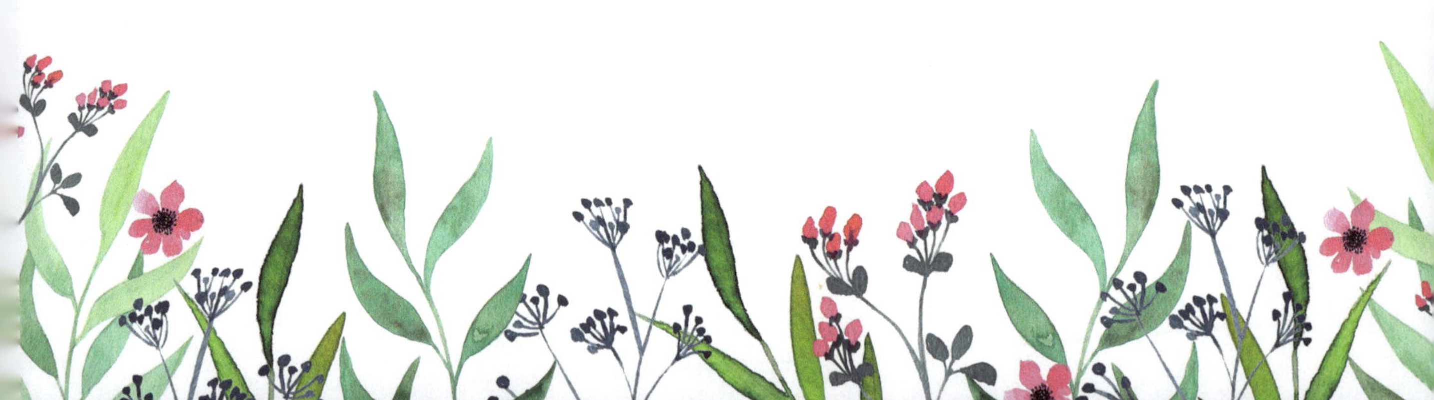

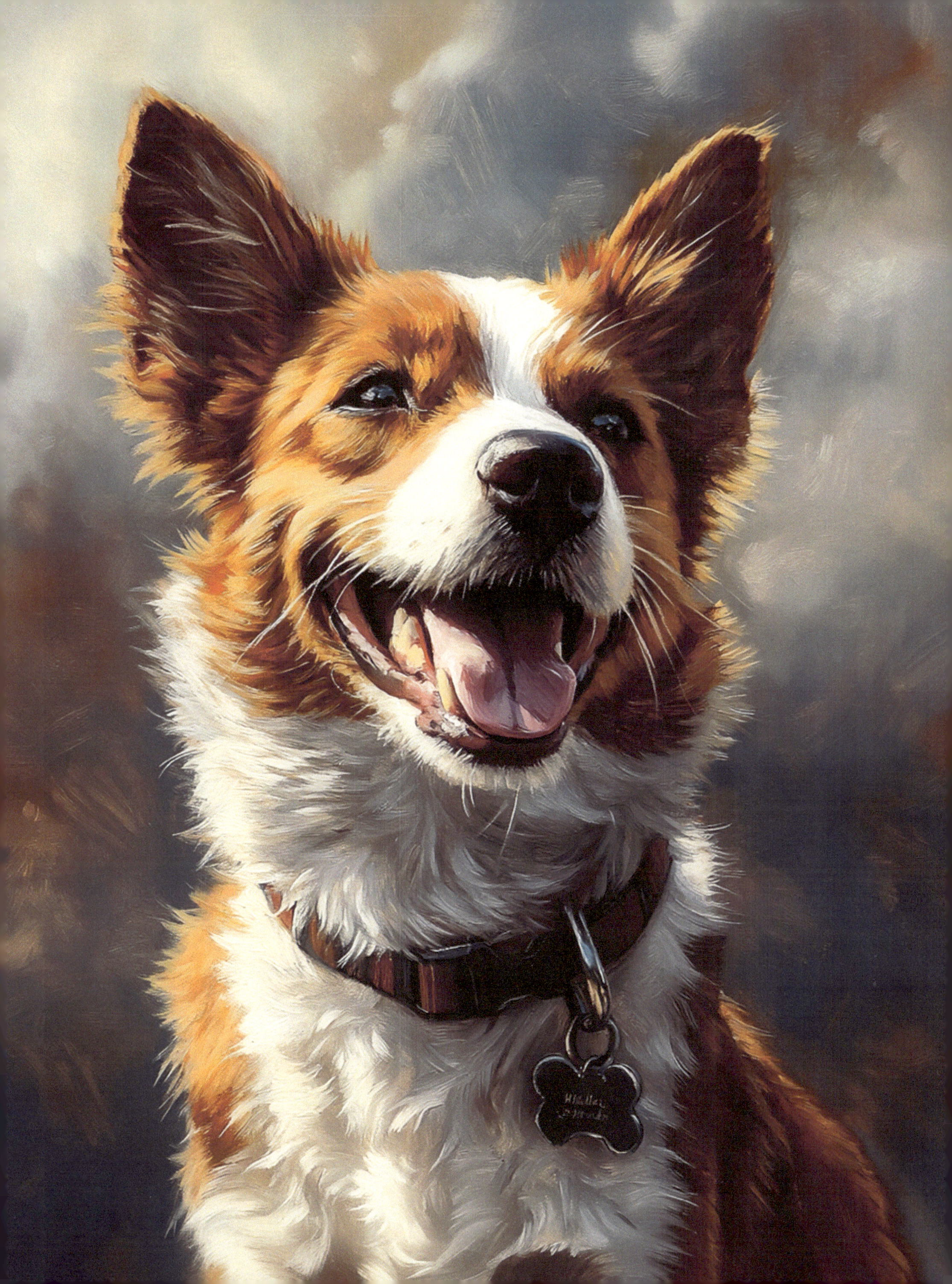

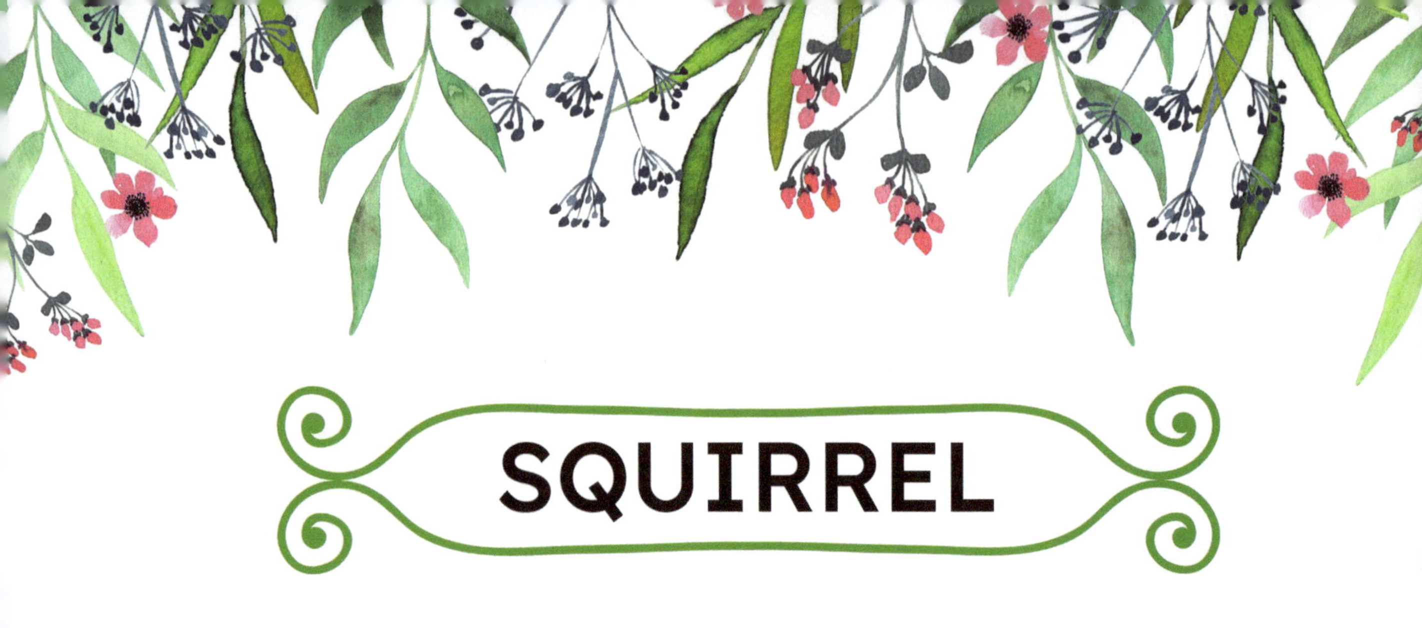

SQUIRREL

Squirrels dart with tails held high,

Chasing leaves that flutter by.

Chirping, leaping branch to branch,

Masters of the nutty dance.

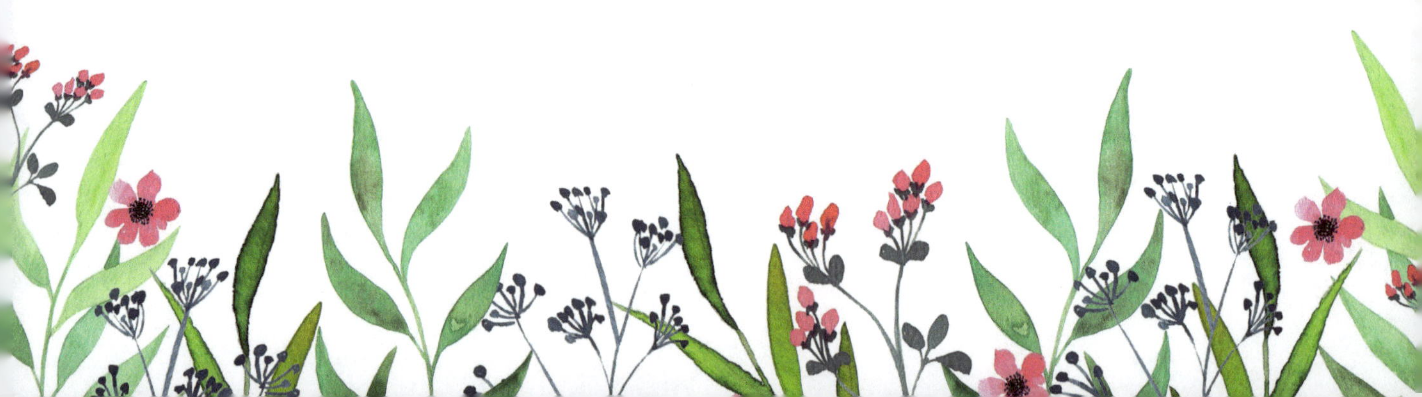

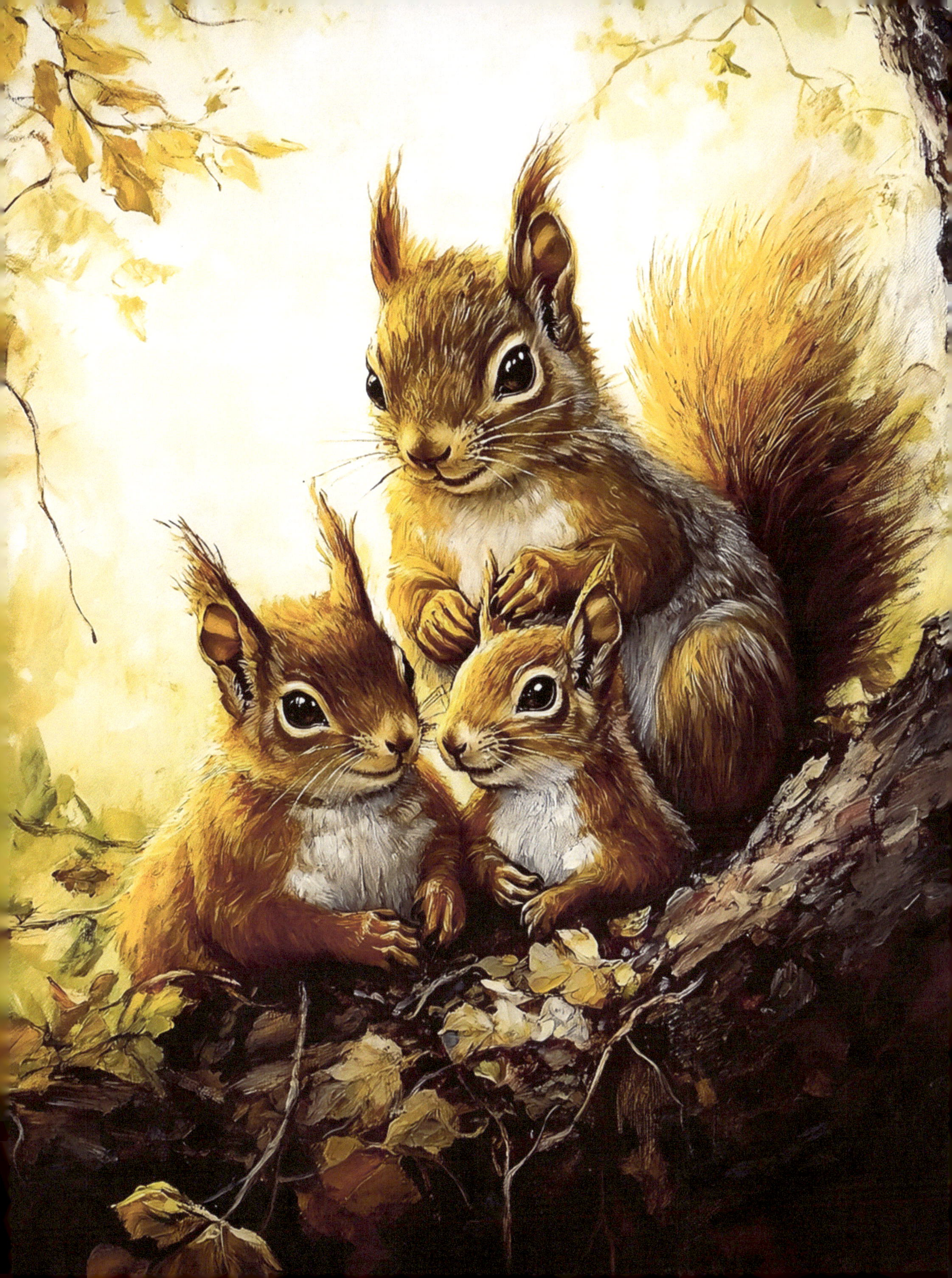

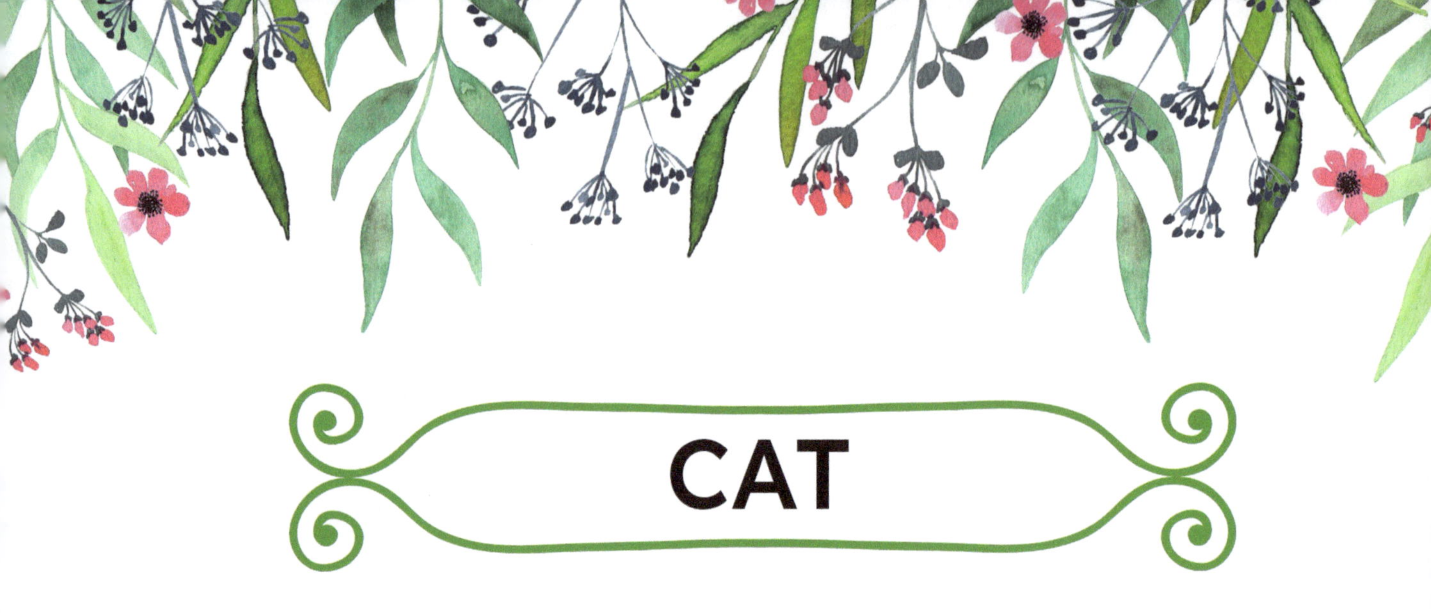

CAT

A mother cat with eyes so bright,

Protects her kitten day and night.

They snuggle close, a cozy heap,

Purring softly as they sleep.

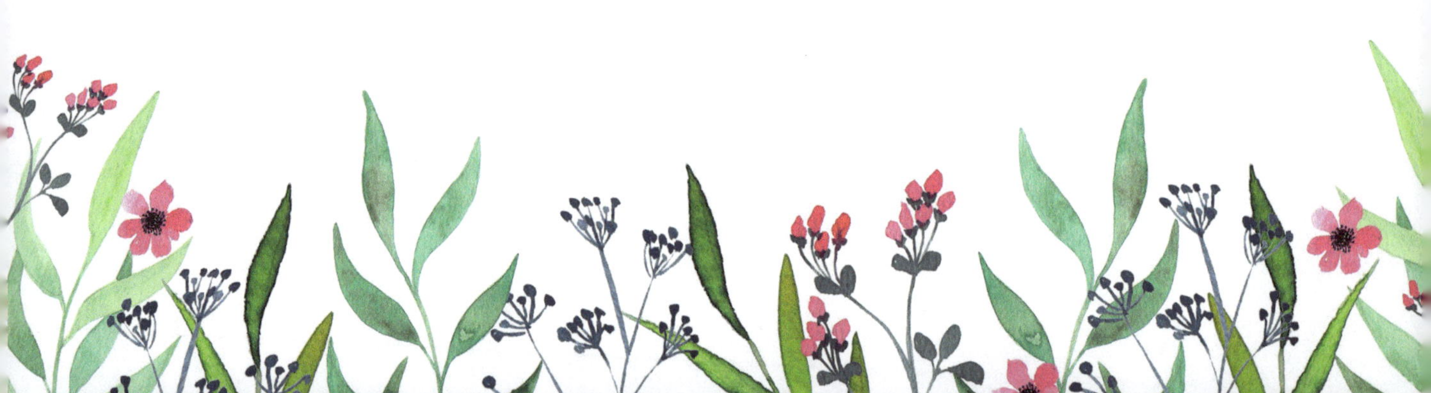

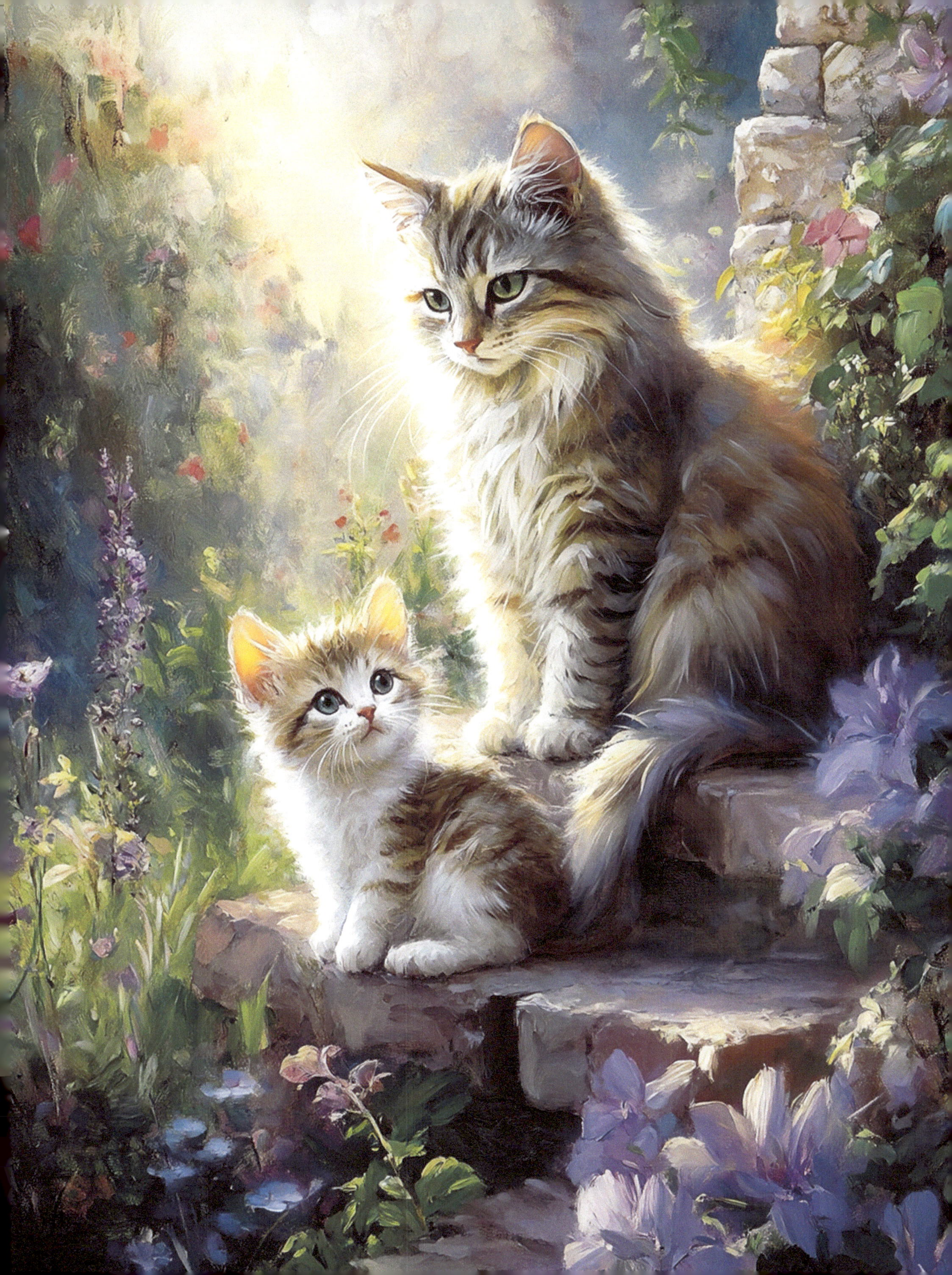

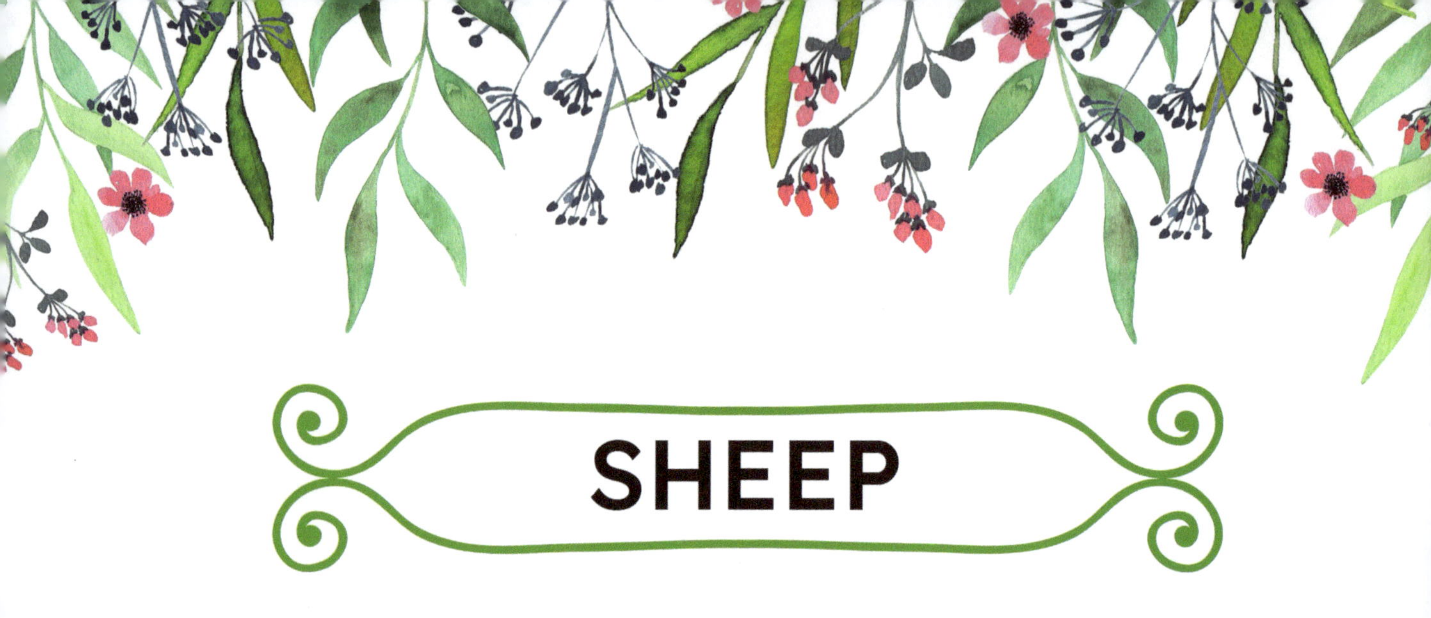

SHEEP

A mother sheep, so soft and white,

Keeps her lamb close, day and night.

They graze together, side by side,

In fields of green, with love and pride.

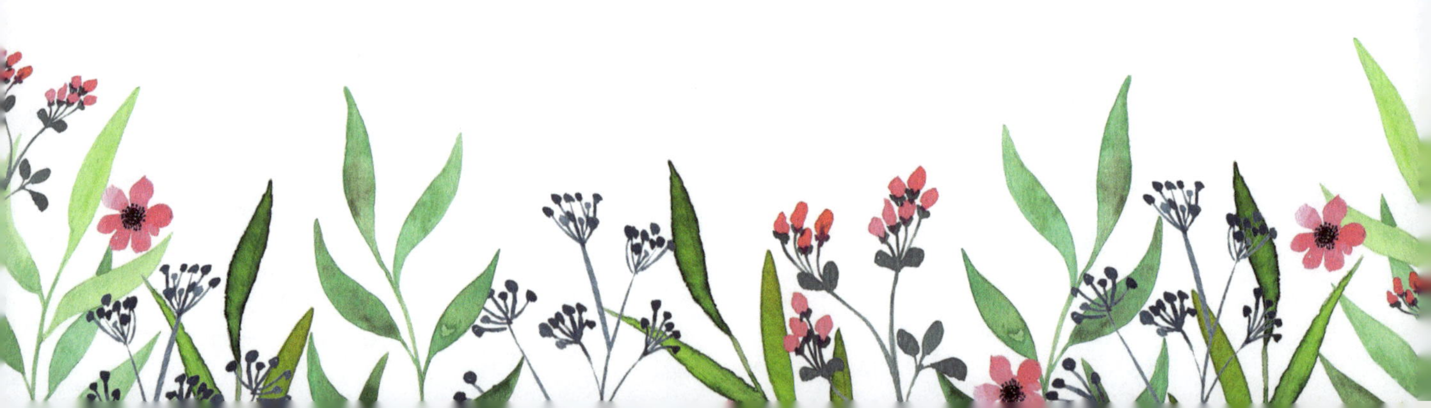

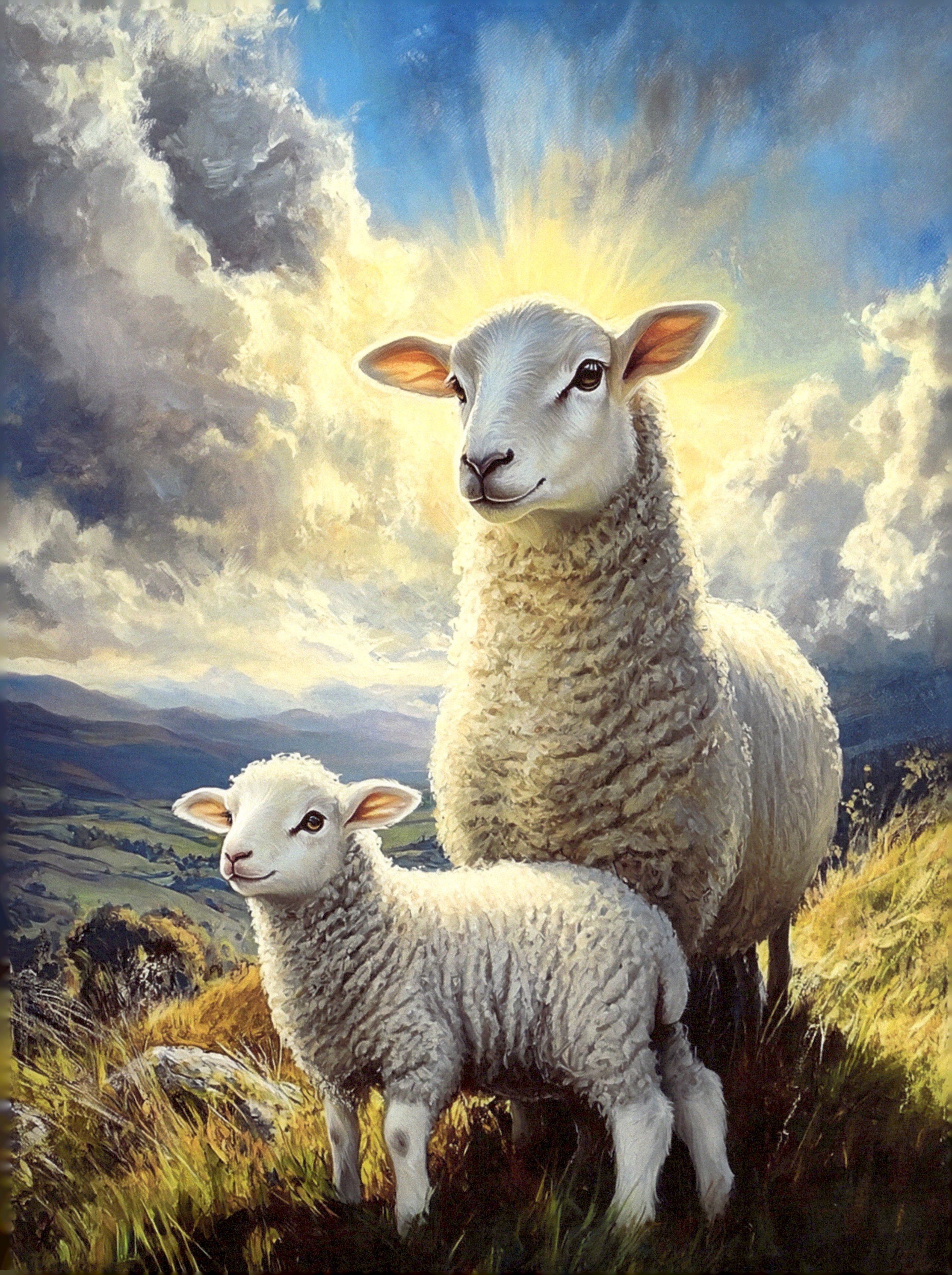